Occupational Therapy

Activities for Practice and Teaching

Occupational Therapy

Activities for Practice and Teaching

ESTELLE B. BREINES, PHD, OTR, FAOTA
Seton Hall University, New Jersey

W
WHURR PUBLISHERS
LONDON AND PHILADELPHIA

First published 2004 by
Whurr Publishers Ltd
19b Compton Terrace, London N1 2UN, England
325 Chestnut Street, Philadelphia PA19106, USA

Reprinted 2005

British Library Cataloguing in Publication Data

A catalogue record for this book is available from the British Library.

ISBN 10- 1 86156 393 0
ISBN 13- 978 1 86156 393 4

Printed and bound in the UK by Athenaeum Press Limited, Gateshead, Tyne & Wear.

Contents

Foreword

The profession of occupational therapy is less than a hundred years old, if a meeting in Clifton Springs, in the USA, is seen as the beginning, yet it is expanding and flourishing all over the world. In 1917, a small group of interested people met at Clifton Springs to found the National Society for the Promotion of Occupational Therapy. Today, the World Federation of Occupational Therapists has fifty-seven member countries and the number is rising steadily.

If success can be measured in terms of growth and expansion, then occupational therapy is a successful profession. This is surely due to the pragmatic value of a professional group whose main concern is to promote and maintain people's ability to function effectively in the world. What could be more useful?

And yet, occupational therapists sometimes appear to doubt our own worth. Perhaps this is because we work in areas of life that everyone takes for granted until something goes wrong. When Mrs Smith wants to regain her ability to get dressed after a stroke, she needs an occupational therapist. When Mr Brown returns to work after an acute psychotic episode, he may depend on the support of an occupational therapist. However, getting dressed and going to work are ordinary, everyday activities. Not everyone is able to recognise the skills that go into performing these activities and that are required for teaching or maintaining them

The skills of the occupational therapist, although crucial to those clients who receive occupational therapy, are mostly invisible to the rest of the world. Occupational therapists are not invited to address the important health issues of the day on national radio. Our interventions do not make great television drama. Some therapists find it difficult to sustain a commitment to working with activity in the face of the puzzlement or indifference of their colleagues.

What the occupational therapist does looks so simple that the observer might think it is just based on common sense. But this practical approach to addressing the ordinary activities of everyday life is underpinned by a coherent philosophy of practice that is the envy of other professions. It is also supported by an impressive body of theory that is being expanded and refined all the time.

In the past, the occupational therapist's professional self-doubt has perhaps been exacerbated by an incongruity between the grand theories that we have tried to adapt to our practice and our focus on small gains with individual clients. When everyone around us is using medical terminology, it can be hard to take pride in talking about mundane matters such as cooking and childcare. This situation is improving as we develop a specialised vocabulary with which to articulate our concerns, our goals and our methods.

In this book, Estelle Breines has succeeded in capturing both the importance of small gains and the complexity of our apparently simple methods, in language that is appropriate to occupational therapy. She describes her collection of meditations on the therapeutic use and value of activity as 'often warm and fuzzy simple stories'. This phrase does not do justice to the wealth of knowledge, understanding and experience that have made it possible to write in such a way. For example, in describing activities that might be appropriate for autumn (Fall: it's finally in the air) Estelle has drawn on her understanding of activity analysis, cultural appropriateness, individual motivation, activity sequencing, accessible environments, group dynamics, risk management and occupational justice. This apparently unsophisticated description of things to do in the autumn is based, like occupational therapy itself, on complex, high level theories.

The book also incorporates some of Estelle's more overtly philosophical and theoretical papers, reproduced with the permission of the original publishers. These enable the reader to explore in more depth some of the concepts that are touched on in the papers that describe aspects of practice. For example, in the story of Elizabeth (Engaging the mind to help the body overcome illness), Estelle describes how being able to carry out two small activities independently made a major difference to the quality of life of a lady living with severe pain and deformity. In the paper on Understanding 'occupation' as the founders did, she gives us a theoretical framework for understanding how these small achievements could have such a great effect.

Occupational therapists are concerned with the modest, daily activities of ordinary people but we should take care not to confuse modesty with insignificance. For someone with a serious, long-term incapacity, small achievements can be very significant. This important truth permeates the writings in Estelle's book. All the papers have appeared in other publications but it is a joy to see them together in a single collection where they form a coherent account of the interaction between theory and practice in occupational therapy.

Jennifer Creek,
Freelance occupational therapist,
North Yorkshire

Preface

In 1994, E.J. Brown of Merion Publications of Philadelphia, Pennsylvania, invited me to write a series of columns on activity for *Advance for Occupational Therapy*, a small weekly, later monthly, newsprint publication whose primary purpose is classified advertising, but which attracts a large readership for its interesting and up-to-date, sometimes controversial articles on occupational therapy. EJ and I talked about the nature of the columns she wanted from me so I could better understand what she had in mind.

To my way of thinking, occupational therapists have a clear idea of what active occupation entails, and how to use it in practice. Certainly my own education had been full of activities and activity analysis, and my years as a practitioner had given me ample experience. And the colleagues I worked with had this knowledge as well, some from their own education and some perhaps from us having worked together over time.

On the other hand, EJ had observed that in the United States, there seemed to be a shift away from using crafts and other activities in practice, and many younger therapists were uninformed as to how to use them effectively as clinical tools. It was apparent that curricula had changed, as many schools had eliminated crafts from their courses. So as schools changed, and clinics changed, therapy had changed as well.

As I had written a text called *Occupational Therapy Activities from Clay to Computers*, which focused on the use of activities in practice, she thought I might be interested in writing some columns that gave examples of how activity could be used effectively. I agreed to try, and the name 'Activity Notebook' became the title of the column, which still continues to this day.

When I began to write these articles, I never envisioned that I would be writing more than a few columns at best. After all, how many topics were there to write about? But I found myself still writing these often warm and fuzzy simple stories some eight years later. Oddly enough, they obtained a broad readership among US therapists, judging by the many emails and letters I have gotten over the years. In some instances, faculties have contacted me asking for permission to distribute some of the articles to students, which I was pleased to do, given that I use them regularly myself in various classes I teach. Students tend to accept the messages in simple stories more readily than dealing with the abstractions of complex texts.

Now that the number of articles I have written has reached a sizable mass, it seemed a good idea to make them available in one text. I hope you will find them enjoyable reading, and can use them to help to explain to the uninitiated the mysteries of occupation and its applications to health and learning.

What goes round comes round

Originally published in *Advance for Occupational Therapy*, Dec. 12, 1994

Several weeks ago, *ADVANCE* ran a story by assistant editor Claudia Stahl on the Arts in Medicine program at Shands Hospital in Gainesville, FL. It detailed the story of a Florida oncologist's move toward using creative activities with almost all his patients because he believed they are therapeutic. In this issue, I understand, Ms. Stahl will take a closer look at the AIM program, which involves everything from ceramics to weaving in the way of crafts. The program is being hailed and publicized as something 'new' and 'innovative' for a hospital setting. Occupational therapists are not providing the crafts; they are being provided on a volunteer basis by unpaid artists in residence.

Do you know that Mary Reilly once stated that if OT were to disappear as a profession, a new profession would soon emerge with the same characteristics? She never predicted, however, that our profession would be reinvented before its demise. Why is it that other disciplines would see value in the tools that OTs traditionally have held dear, while many OTs have lost their reverence for these same tools?

When I was an undergraduate student at NYU in 1957, it was expected that students would come to the program with a strong interest in handcrafts. In fact, one of the reasons students were attracted to OT was the opportunity to hone their skills in crafts while learning to use them in therapy. The curriculum included courses in ceramics, woodworking, metal crafts, weaving and other crafts. At the same time, we took anatomy, physiology, kinesiology, neurology, psychology, physical and mental conditions, and courses which taught us to splint, adapt equipment, analyze activities and use them in treatment.

Crafts were our tools; we learned to understand the world through them; we learned to use them with patients of all sorts; we had the skills we needed — and we knew who we were. I can remember as a student marching the halls of New York Hospital with a huge picnic hamper on my arm, filled with a selection of items I might need as I went from patient to patient. Whether I was dealing with patients with Hodgkins disease, poliomyelitis, lupus erythematosis, or brachial plexus injury, there was always something appropriate in that basket: spools of leather lacing, needles, yarns, scissors, glue, and doubtless many other things. I can remember better how heavy the basket was.

From that time to this we have seen many changes in health care. Some conditions we treated in the past are no longer seen, while new ones have taken their place; but I suspect the changes in occupational therapy modalities are more related to our unwillingness to identify with mundane things. We sought to characterize ourselves as scientists, while the arts that were special to us diminished in importance.

Peloquin recently suggested we return to the definition we used to use, highlighting 'the art and science' of occupational therapy. Not only is practice an art, but we have tools that are arts, and it is to these arts that we must return, or others will come to use them.

In January I will begin a monthly column in *ADVANCE*, dedicated to resurfacing issues about the use of creative activities in practice. For many young therapists, such activities remain a mystery. Beyond the skills needed to use them competently, therapists need to come to value these activities and perform them with pride. If other professions can see the value in our tools, we, too, must recognize that value. It's time to bring our skills and our identity back together by initiating a dialogue about these ideas of such fundamental importance to our profession.

The Activity Notebook will deal with the use of activities in practice. I plan to discuss the integration of mind and body in purposeful activity; activity analysis and grading of activity; case studies in all areas of practice; teaching methods; purchasing, budgeting and billing issues; cultural relevance and regional preferences; and others.

If you are experienced, please share your ideas with me: if you are not let me know what you want to learn, and I'll try to meet your needs. Growing a dialogue can help us save this important part of our professional repertoire for ourselves.

Times have certainly changed, but they appear to be changing back. It seems that true concepts are timeless.

Introduction

This book is divided into ten chapters which cover a series of topics of interest to occupational therapists. The articles were written, however, in a random order and the organization was undertaken much later. The disorganized approach to the writing is reflective of a problem the profession has in explaining itself as we move back and forth, to and from reductionistic and holistic conceptualizations. These articles were written in an attempt to simplify some complex notions that arose from a study of the underlying philosophical principles that influenced the development of the profession, in order to make them more palatable for readers who would rather focus on less abstract thoughts.

I write with an American bias that I request the reader to forgive. Aside from the fact that the articles originally were written by an American for an American audience, my bias comes from my belief that our profession was instigated by strong influences from the mental hygiene movement which in turn was influenced by the American pragmatists John Dewey, William James, Charles Peirce and George Herbert Mead. In turn, their ideas were driven by the relational notions of Hegel in conjunction with the evolutionary precepts of Charles Darwin.

The pragmatists adopted the notions of time, development and evolution as concepts of change evident in human behavior and experience. They departed from a prevailing notion of truth as absolute, affirming the relevance of objectivity and subjectivity in understanding human endeavor. Each of these scholars applied these ideas to their own specialized areas of study. Peirce's notions, the most abstract, were applied by James to the study of psychology, by Mead to the study of sociology and by Dewey to the study of education, in which he advanced the notion of learning by doing.

These ideas were promulgated widely at the University of Chicago and elsewhere in the United States and influenced members of the Illinois and National Mental Hygiene Societies, whose names may be familiar to readers.

Among these persons of prominence were Adolf Meyer, Eleanor Clarke Slagle, Rabbi Emil Gustave Hirsch, Julia Lathrop and Jane Addams, all foundational figures for American occupational therapy. Hirsch and Lathrop founded the Chicago School for Civics and Philanthropy, the first occupational therapy school, at Addams' Hull House where Slagle and Mary Potter Brooks Meyer (Adolf Meyer's wife) studied occupational therapy. It was here that learning through doing was adopted as the profession's foundational belief.

Drawing on evolutionary themes, pragmatism, which is a phenomenological philosophical movement, advanced the concept of adaptation that was also adopted by occupational therapy. The pragmatists focused on the ideas that mind and body are inseparable and that the individual contributes to society, just as society contributes to the individual. Occupational therapy established its belief in bringing people to their highest levels of functioning so they could become contributing members of society. The founders of the National Society for the Promotion of Occupational Therapy, later the American Occupational Therapy Association, demonstrated the application of these ideas across the various disorders of mind and body.

In time, these abstract ideas were set aside by the occupational therapy profession. Attention was largely focused on the mundane, practical aspects of living as occupational therapists opened the door to the acceptance of common sense as a guide for behavior. Yet, in time, the profession again looked for philosophical explanations for what we inherently know and experience.

In an attempt to meet this need, I, along with others, began to study and analyze our profession's origins and organizing beliefs. As I studied the ideas of the pragmatists, I tried to formulate a comprehensive model that featured ideas held by occupational therapists, describing this model as occupational genesis. Occupational genesis describes the interactions among egocentric elements (mind and body), exocentric elements (time and space) and consensual elements (social factors such as relationships, language, roles, regulations), and the changes in these interactions over the course of time. For example, infants move randomly with primitive cognitive abilities (egocentric), surrounded by cribs and mobile toys (exocentric), relating to caretakers in dependent roles (consensual). As development progresses, physical and mental skills develop (egocentric), the toys and environments of childhood (exocentric) alter and relationships with siblings, friends and family grow (consensual). As aging progresses, each of these elements and their interactions change.

This model also applies to the understanding of cultural development.

Drawing from Dewey's work in the Laboratory School at the University of Chicago, we can observe that the knowledge base and skills of individuals and the artifacts of cultures change over time, influencing and being influenced by social relationships and the activities in which one engages.

Human evolution is driven by the relationships among egocentric, exocentric and consensual elements. In each time period and in each geographic environment, humans drew upon their physical and mental capacities, in conjunction with the tangible features of their environments, in collaboration with those in their society. From this idea, the model of occupational technology emerged. Occupational technology is based on the premise that human beings have been technological creatures from the beginning of pre-history to the modern era, in the same way that occupational therapists have been technologists from their inception to today.

Occupational genesis focuses on the relational and developmental nature of humans. Occupational technology focuses on the technological features of that development. Both are derivatives of the pragmatists' beliefs, organized to create models for occupational therapists to use in clinical practice, education and research.

The reader is urged to read original and interpretive texts to better understand than I can explain what the pragmatists offered. Toward this end, I suggest a list of papers and books to help guide your reading. And in keeping with the ordinary things that ordinary people express themselves through, I offer the simple articles that follow.

Suggested additional readings

Breines EB (1986) Origins and Adaptations: A Philosophy of Practice. Lebanon, NJ: Geri-Rehab.

Breines EB (1992) Rabbi Emil G. Hirsch: ethical philosopher and founding figure of occupational therapy. Israel Journal of Occupational Therapy 1: E1–E10.

Breines EB (1995) Occupational Therapy Activities from Clay to Computers: Theory and Practice. Philadelphia: F.A. Davis.

Dewey J (1916) Democracy and Education: An Introduction to the Philosophy of Education. Toronto: Collier Macmillan.

Dewey J (1929) The Quest for Certainty: A Study of the Relation of Knowledge and Action. New York: Minton, Balch & Co.

Mayhew KC, Edwards AC (1936) The Dewey School: the Lab School of the University of Chicago. 1896–1903. New York: Appleton-Century.

Serrett KD (1985) Another look at occupational therapy's history: paradigm or pair of hands? Occupational Therapy in Mental Health 5(3): 1–31.

Understanding 'occupation' as the founders did

Originally published in *British Journal of Occupational Therapy*, Nov. 1995, 58(11): 458–60

Abstract

The term 'occupation' is both ambiguous and encompassing. This term was adopted by the founders of the profession as a means of incorporating a variety of perspectives on the profession. Interrelating concepts deriving from pragmatism and the mental hygiene movement offer a rationale for understanding occupation. Terms used to describe occupation are egocentricity (mind/body elements), exocentricity (time/space elements) and consensuality (social elements). The integration of these aspects in occupation offers an explanation for the holism advanced by the profession at its outset and today.

Introduction

The literature of occupational therapy repeatedly calls for the definition and accurate use of terms. Darnell and Heater (1994) reiterate this call, in this case urging the explicit use of the term 'occupation' in lieu of terms such as activity. They ground their argument in Nelson's (1988) work, which defines occupation as 'the relationship between occupational form and occupational performance' (p. 633).

Defining occupation, just like defining occupational therapy, seems to be a process in which occupational therapists repeatedly engage (Christiansen, 1994; Mosey, 1981). Although the Representative Assembly of the American Occupational Therapy Association (AOTA) has recently adopted new and comprehensive definitions of various terms essential to the profession, including occupation (Position Paper on Occupation, 1995, unpublished), there is no reason to believe that the last word has been written about this topic of critical concern to the profession. Therefore, new perspectives on this word of such importance to the profession may be useful for helping therapists to explain themselves and their work to patients and colleagues, and may serve as a basis for study and research.

The term occupation has been used to describe various models and concepts. These include occupational behaviour (Reilly, 1974), human occupation (Kielhofner and Burke, 1980), occupational performance (Llorens, 1979; Mosey, 1981), occupational genesis (Breines, 1990), occupational science (Clark et al., 1991) and occupational adaptation (Schkade and Schultz, 1992).

Certainly, the term occupation is used freely to describe various conceptual organizations, and appears to mean many different things. Darnell and Heater (1994) are correct to suggest the clarification of the term occupation, and to invite the expanded use of this term to characterize the profession which carries its name. In response, this article frames the discussion in terms deriving from foundation philosophical and historical sources.

At the outset

This author believes that, at the outset of the profession, the term occupation was deliberately selected because of both its ambiguity and its comprehensiveness. An attempt is made to demonstrate this through extrapolation from historical and philosophical evidence, because one is limited to post hoc interpretation when the original sources neglected to offer explicit answers to questions that emerge long after the witnesses are gone.

At the outset, there was considerable discussion about naming the profession. After numerous suggestions, such as 'reeducation' and 'reconstruction', were rejected by one or another of the founders in vigorous debate, the term occupational therapy was selected (Barton, c. 1914–17; Dunton, c. 1916–17; Licht, 1967; Slagle, c. 1916–17). Occupation appears to have been a word that the founders could agree upon, possibly because it held various meanings and could serve as a mediating term. To find a common word for a profession that synthesized many views was critical, because the profession was founded by a number of individuals who saw the value of occupation in different arenas of practice. Among these were Barton (1919) in sheltered work and physical rehabilitation; Dunton (1918) and Slagle (1914) in mental health; Kidner (c. 1917) in tuberculosis; and Tracy (1918) in medical illness.

Many of these individuals were influenced by the mental hygiene movement. This movement, which originated in the USA around the turn of the century, was recognized for its efforts in social activism (Cohen, 1983). The mental hygiene movement had many members in common with the Arts and Crafts movement, and had many principles in common. Many of the foundational figures of occupation therapy, including Adolf Meyer and Eleanor Clarke Slagle, were affiliated with the National Mental Hygiene Society or the Illinois Mental Hygiene Society (Breines, 1986a).

The mental hygiene movement was influenced by the philosophy of pragmatism expounded at the University of Chicago. Pragmatism is a phenomenological philosophy which focuses on the relationships among individuals, their artifacts and environments and their societies, as represented by their actions in personal and interpersonal well-being. John Dewey, a principal proponent of pragmatism, is recognized for the concept widely known as 'learning through doing'.

Both the Chicago School for Civics and Philanthropy, where Slagle studied occupational therapy, and the Henry B Faville School of Occupational Therapy, where she later taught, were located at Hull House in Chicago, where pragmatism was taught by John Dewey and Julia Lathrop (Addams, 1910). The Faville School functioned under the sponsorship of the Illinois Mental Hygiene Society. And it was at the University of Chicago that Adolf Meyer (1950) taught and had collegial relationships with John

Dewey and George Herbert Mead, foundational philosophers of pragmatism. Here, social activism and pragmatism were united, and built foundations for occupational therapy (Breines, 1986a; Serrett, 1985a, 1985b).

Pragmatism speaks to the interaction of the mind and body of individuals with their tangible and social environments by means of active occupation (Dewey, 1916; Mead, 1932, 1938). This relational belief system, structured in concepts of time, evolution, history and development, can serve as a model for understanding the term occupation and other terms stemming from the same root.

Three distinct concepts

'Occupation' can be described according to three distinct but interrelating concepts; egocentric, exocentric and consensual. These three concepts derive from the model of occupational genesis (see Figure 1; Breines, 1990, 1995), and are grounded in pragmatism. Occupational genesis defines *egocentric* as all aspects of mind and body; exocentric as all aspects of time and space; and *consensual* as all social phenomena such as roles, rules and language. Consistent with the relational aspects of pragmatism, these three concepts, egocentricity, exocentricity and consensuality, and their components – mind, body, time, space and others such as social influences – are in constant flux and interact throughout life in the performance of life's tasks.

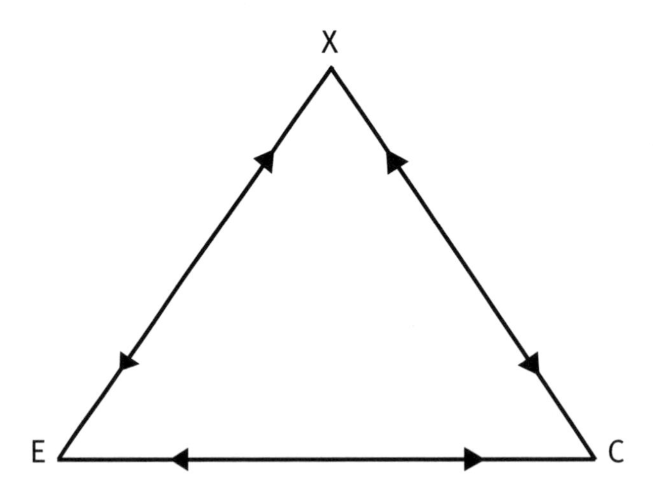

Figure 1: Egocentric (E), exocentric (X), and consensual (C) elements influence one another. The relationships among these elements are represented by the lines. Occupational therapy changes these relationships by influencing (adapting) any or all of these elements: mind/body, time/space, or social interactions.
Source: Breines (1995). Copyright © 1995, FA Davis.

Three major concepts are revealed when analyzing the term occupation. These concepts are:

1. *To be occupied*, representing the *egocentric* aspect. When one is occupied, one is engaged both in mind and in body, sometimes simultaneously, sometimes alternatively. When performing a task, mind and body integrate. When the mind is occupied, the body performs. When the body is occupied, the mind is distracted or engaged. These interactive phenomena are called upon in practice and underlie the concept of goal-directed activity. Occupational therapy is focused primarily on the education of mind and/or body toward health.
2. *To occupy*, representing the *exocentric* aspect. When engaged in tasks, one occupies space and occupies time; one is interacting with these elements of the environment, while these elements themselves interact. That is, the individual learns to adapt to the world and/or the environment is adapted to the individual. Both of these perspectives on adaptation are reflected in practice, as in the use of wheelchairs and splints, and in learning skills used in self-care, work and play. Adaptation, whether spatial or temporal, is a fundamental tool and expectation of practice.
3. *Occupation*, representing the *consensual* aspect. This third aspect is often described in terms of vocation or work, but also represents interactive play or other endeavors in which one collaborates, competes or otherwise engages with or for others in socially responsible behaviors. Play-based therapies, activity group process, work hardening, sheltered workshops and homemaking training, all aspects of occupational therapy practice, fall under this rubric.

Addressing the meaning of occupational therapy

These three uses of the term occupation together address the meaning of occupational therapy as suggested by our founders, and as understood today. The human being engages all these elements – mind, body, time, space and others – in performing life's tasks, and practice considers them all, using each element to affect each other element in the pursuit of health. These fundamental concepts prevail regardless of clinical population, but different areas of practice emphasize different elements. 'Psych. OTs' may emphasize the mind while 'phys.dis. OTs' may emphasize the body, but both consider each other element as it applies to their patients. All therapists use the physical and social environments to effect change.

The diverse ways in which occupation can be defined suggests that this term is extraordinarily comprehensive. Moreover, precisely because of this comprehensiveness, occupation has evaded unique definition.

The founders' selection of the term occupation to describe the profession was not incidental. Considerable argument was entered into before the name of our profession was selected (Barton, c. 1914–17; Licht, 1967; Slagle, c. 1916–17). Rather, this author believes that the term 'occupation' was ultimately decided upon to mean all of the elements described above, in part and in whole, if not explicitly, then in terms of its compatibility with the various beliefs of the founders. Furthermore, this holistic interpretation may be the reason that the term has been retained as the profession's identity, despite recurring reports of discomfort with it (Marmer, 1994; ADVANCE Staff, 1994).

Were the profession to dissociate itself from any of the three elements of occupation cited above, it would no longer be the profession it has aspired to be. In the absence of any one element – mind, body, time, space and others – we could not be who we are, nor practice as we do in the holistic breadth of practice. The term occupation encapsulates all aspects of who we are as a profession because it represent the comprehensiveness that identifies us. What brilliance the founders demonstrated in arriving at this identity for the profession!

Conclusion

This analysis is consistent with the profession's foundational philosophy, and is consistent with practice in all its elements, at our origin as well as today. This interpretation may help therapists better to comprehend diverse features of their profession that have sometimes appeared to be in conflict, while recognizing the position of these separate elements in regard to the holism of the profession. Furthermore, this analysis, in addition to other descriptions and uses of the term occupation, affirms the comprehensiveness with which this holistic profession and its philosophy hold.

Rabbi Emil Gustave Hirsch: ethical philosopher and founding figure of occupational therapy

Originally published in *Israel Journal of Occupational Therapy* 1992 1(1): E1–E9

Abstract

Rabbi Hirsch is identified in several sources as a founder of the Chicago School of Civics and Philanthropy, the first school of Occupational Therapy. Hirsch's relations are traced to the Chicago School of Civics and Philanthropy and Addams, Julia Lathrop, John Dewey, George Herbert Mead, Adolf Meyer, and the Baltimore community. Hirsch's religious and ethical philosophy are analyzed and correlated with principles of pragmatism and occupational therapy, in which enablement is advanced as being of mutual benefit to the individual and society.

Introduction

> *Julia Lathrop and Rabbi Hirsch founded the first school of Occupational Therapy at the Chicago School for Civics and Philanthropy. (Dunton, 1915)*

This statement was made in 1915 in a book by Dr William Rush Dunton, Jr., one of the founders of the National Society for the Promotion of Occupational Therapy (NSPOT), the forerunner of the American Occupational Therapy Association (AOTA). Dunton's statement is repeated in several secondary sources (Brunyate, 1958; Licht, 1967), but is not elaborated on, and does not reveal Lathrop and Hirsch's reasons for establishing the school. This brief statement is the *only* indication that Hirsch was an individual of significance to Occupational Therapy. No other mention of Hirsch appears in Occupational Therapy literature, and no mention of Occupational Therapy appears in Hirsch's papers.

Historical associations

While there is no direct reference, either in archival material or secondary sources as to Hirsch's specific purpose with regard to Occupational Therapy, the literature reveals an abundance of sources from which his ideals can be extrapolated, and the case can be made that he held similar beliefs to those of his colleagues and contemporaries.

At the turn of the century, the faculty at the University of Chicago included: John Dewey (1916) and George Herbert Mead (1932), the famous pragmatist philosophers; Hirsch, himself a philosopher, educator and religious leader; Jane Addams (1910), the great social activist of Hull House; Oscar Triggs (1902), a founder of the Arts and Crafts Movement in the United States; and Adolf Meyer (1922), the renowned neurologist and psychiatrist.

The philosophy of pragmatism, based upon Darwin's theme of evolution and Hegel's theme of relationship or dialectic, was prevalent here. Hirsch's biographer and son (Hirsch, 1968) reports that Hirsch, as well as Dewey, were students of Hegel's dialectics, as was Hirsch's father before him. Pragmatism's philosophy of time, also expressed as evolution and history, was a critical theme of the University. This theme found its application in many veins of thought and action. These concepts were analyzed from many perspectives, each scholar particularizing these ideas to their own interests.

The universal theme to which these scholars ascribed was the relationship of the individual to society and the benefit of each to the other as a phenomenon needed for growth, change and adaptation in a positive direction. They recognized this relationship as significant to health. They believed that society's health is dependent upon the welfare of the individual, and the health of the individual relates to the welfare of society. The mental hygiene movement took its purpose from this premise. Asserting these beliefs, the mental hygiene movement counted Dewey, James, Addams, Lathrop, Meyer, and Hirsch as members (Cohen, 1983; Slagle, c. 1917). For them, education and health were one.

The relationship between these individuals and Occupational Therapy's founding figures has been neglected until recent times (Breines, 1986b, 1989a), but the relationship existed (Lidz, 1985; Serrett, 1985c). However, the position of Hirsch is most obscure, since the only reference to him is the brief and repeated statement by Dunton in 1915. This paper will review Emil Hirsch's history, analyze selected writings of Hirsch for their correlation with the pragmatic perspective, and attempt to demonstrate Hirsch's influence upon Occupational Therapy.

Emil Gustave Hirsch

Dr Emil Gustave Hirsch, rabbi at Congregation Sinai in Chicago, was a prominent leader of American Reform Judaism during the period surrounding the turn of the century (*Encyclopedia Judaica*, 1978). Hirsch lived from 1851 to 1923. Coming from a family of renowned rabbis, he followed his father and uncle in that calling, and was ordained as a Reform rabbi. Rejecting an Orthodox heritage, as did his father before him, Hirsch was described as a militant (Hirsch, 1968; GLB, 1935).

While a brilliant scholar (Hirsch was conversant in 17 languages, and acknowledged leader in the Chicago and national religious and social communities), few of Hirsch's personal papers remain for us. Hirsch's principles can be discerned from the small collection of items held at the American Jewish Archives – Jewish Institute of Religion in Cincinnati. While these papers contain no direct references to Occupational Therapy, they reveal Hirsch's concern for the community's health and welfare, his interest in active occupation, and his role in developing a manual training school for disadvantaged youngsters in the Chicago community (Hirsch, 1968), and his relationship with other foundational figures of the profession. Addams' (1935) book, *My Friend Julia Lathrop*, confirms Hirsch's involvement with Lathrop in a number of social projects. Their concern for the disadvantaged is revealed by their active involvement with numerous agencies devoted to the care of children, the elderly and the handicapped. From these and other limited sources, Hirsch's guiding principles are revealed, and from these sources one can extrapolate his persuasions.

He reminds 'the mighty of their obligations to the weak and stirs the weak to efforts to conquer their weakness', demanding not only attention from those who are able, but effort from the afflicted in resolving their dysfunction. He speaks of the 'healthy realism' of dealing with 'actualities' (Hirsch, 1892, p. 2962) toward meeting society's needs, thereby addressing the reality of daily life.

It is in the theme of 'tzedakah' that Hirsch's view of ethics is revealed. He characterizes 'tzedakah' in terms of enablement, as opposed to 'giving'. This principle of enablement, viewed by Hirsch as a religious theme, was described by Dewey and Addams as a social obligation. It was adopted through Hirsch's and Lathrop's offices as the Occupational Therapy premise at the Chicago School of Civics and Philanthropy, the first school to teach such principles. The Chicago School of Civics and Philanthropy, Hull House, and Dewey's Laboratory School were concurrent entities, and were each based on uniform principles (Breines, 1986a, 1986b).

Hirsch had other perspectives from which he viewed adaptation and occupation. Hirsch felt that God mandated one day of rest every seventh day, and the specific day of rest was not the pertinent issue of the commandment. Rather, Hirsch viewed six days of labor as mankind's vital and obligatory contribution to society, so it was the active, albeit unmentioned aspect of the commandment which was significant. Work was a religious commitment. The relationship between work and rest, principles also addressed by Meyer, were foundational concepts for Hirsch. Hirsch adapted the pragmatic premises of adaptation and active occupation in accord with current social needs and welfare, demonstrating this principle for modern religion and society.

Hirsch's beliefs melded well with the Quaker principles advanced by Jane Addams. The health of the individual and the community through action in collaborative benefit was long a principle of Quakers and Jews alike.

Hirsch and Addams shared the podium many times and at many places. They were allied in their beliefs and were frequently invited to speak on social issues which concerned them both. It was at Addam's Hull House that the Chicago School of Civics and Philanthropy flowered. The principles of active occupation and adaptation promoted by Dewey and adopted by Hirsch, Lathrop and Addams were taught there to its students Eleanor Clarke Slagle and Mary Potter Brooks Meyer. It was at Hull House that the Faville School of Occupational Therapy was established, and Slagle later taught, a school founded and supported by the Chicago Mental Hygiene Society (Breines, 1986a, 1986b; Slagle, c. 1917).

The memorial document published by the Chicago Council of Jewish Women upon Hirsch's death ascribes four distinct principles to him (Cowen, 1923). These are identified as Religion, Education, Civic Cooperation and Philanthropy. While no mention was made of the Chicago School of Civics and Philanthropy, it too advanced these latter themes. The underlying principle of the first school for Occupational Therapy was to benefit society by enabling individuals to take their role in contributing to that society. Emil Gustave Hirsch was undoubtedly instrumental in establishing these concepts there, the ancient Judaic traditions of education and study in the pursuit of knowledge, of adaptation to a changing world, of tzedakah, and of strong concern for community and individual, enabling growth through activity, contributed to the development of a profession which retains these principles. For Hirsch, grading of abilities in a constant striving for heightened knowledge and heightened contribution to society, by improving the ability of individuals to perform in their own and their society's behalf, was an ethical and religious issue. His interests in issues fundamental to Occupational Therapy appear to indicate Hirsch's motives in regard to founding Occupational Therapy's first school (Breines, 1989a).

Hirsch's heritage

More remarkable than the connections between this remarkable man and a profession that has not acknowledged his role in its founding, nor can be certain of that role, is that despite the dearth of documentation regarding Hirsch's influences upon the profession, his principles guide Occupational Therapists to this day. They retain the principles of adaptation and development in a theme of occupational genesis (Breines, 1990), advancing the ability of individuals to contribute actively to their own needs and those of their society in work, play and leisure, in every era. Occupational Therapists continue to apply the principles to which Hirsch ascribed, in a practice based on ethics which have meaning in the real world, even as it changes. If Hirsch is right in stipulating that, 'Genesis is a divine poem whose last has not yet been written' (Hirsch, 1892, p. 2960), occupational therapy's role in that transition is clear.

Acknowledgements

Appreciation is extended to Rabbi Edward J. Sukol for identifying Rabbi Emil G. Hirsch's connections to the Chicago community; and to Fannie Zelcher, American Jewish Archives – Jewish Institute of Religion, Cincinnati, Ohio for her assistance with the Hirsch papers.

Pragmatism as a foundation for occupational therapy curricula

Originally published in *American Journal of Occupational Therapy* Aug. 1987, 41(8): 522–5)

Abstract

This paper shows that the founders of occupational therapy adhered to the philosophy of pragmatism. A structure for curriculum design based on this philosophy is presented.

It is proposed that clarifying our foundational philosophy to students by means of this structure would enhance their synthesis of occupational therapy concepts.

Curriculum design is an ongoing concern for even the long-established occupational therapy program. Curricula are under constant review. As a result, educational programs have exhibited considerable change over the years (Colman, 1984). In particular, two changes in occupational therapy curricula are of significance. Early occupational therapy education emphasized activities; a shift occurred during the 1960s when a greater emphasis was placed on scientific content. The inclusion of sensory integration (Ayres, 1975) and neurodevelopmental content material (Bobath, 1979; Rood, 1962; Voss, Ionta, and Myers, 1985) are such examples. The second change occurred toward the late 1970s when additional emphasis was placed on issues of theory development and philosophic content (Kielhofner, 1982; Mosey, 1970; Yerxa, 1979).

One reason for these two major changes may have been feelings of professional inadequacy. The more 'scientific' and 'professional' a discipline becomes, the more status and recognition it receives and the more easily it can obtain reimbursement for its services. As professionalization became the goal (Yerxa, 1967; Fidler, 1979), occupational therapy, as well as other professions, placed greater emphasis on scientific theoretical content to gain recognition and status.

As curriculum changes took place, the original values were not always retained in modern education, except in the form of assumptions. The themes which early occupational therapists held dear were no longer understood and therefore undervalued. Early precepts were considered inadequate for delivering practice. Scientific rationales were sought; new theories were developed and debated. Disparities between the old assumptions and the new theories created a conflict and caused anxiety for the profession, akin to the Kuhnian crises Kielhofner (1982) describes. The profession's foundational philosophy and the new emphasis on science were not synthesized. The stress caused by this lack of a synthesis is reflected in the various and sometimes conflicting definitions and models used to describe the profession.

One reason that occupational therapy has suffered from the lack of a strong, professional identity is that its foundational principles were never clearly defined, not even by the founders of the profession. The foundational beliefs of the profession were not clearly stated in the early literature. The only exception is the paper published by Meyer in 1922, but even Meyer's paper offers no citations and therefore no support for his position.

The story of the history of occupational therapy is usually told as though it began in 1917 at a curative workshop in New York State. However, occupational therapy as a profession was influenced by the intellectual and social ideas of the times and by national and worldwide events such as immigration, war, and the industrial revolution (Breines, 1986a, 1986b).

These influences led to the development of the first school for the instruction of occupation as a therapeutic modality (Dunton, 1915), The Chicago School of Civics and Philanthropy (CSCP), in 1908. Associated with the CSCP were Emil G. Hirsch, Julia Lathrop, Eleanor Clarke Slagle, and Mary Potter Brooks Meyer, the wife of Adolf Meyer. These leaders were influenced by ideas from the philosophy of pragmatism.

Adherents to pragmatism included Charles Peirce, the philosopher; William James, the psychologist and philosopher; George Herbert Mead, the sociologist and philosopher; and John Dewey, the educator, philosopher, and social activist. Mead and Dewey were faculty members at the University of Chicago.

There is evidence to suggest that ideas of the pragmatists were shared by the early advocates of occupational therapy. Adolf Meyer was a colleague and friend of Mead and Dewey; they all served on the faculty of the University of Chicago. Meyer also met James while working and teaching in Massachusetts. He credits these scholars for many of the concepts he expresses throughout his extensive writings (Winters, 1952, vol. 1, p. 246; vol. 2 pp. 215, 228; Vol. 3, pp. 64, 102, 462; Vol. 4, pp. 102, 242, 469, 482).

The University of Chicago was a center for study and practice based on pragmatic principles. Formal and informal relationships were developed with the community. Dewey's Laboratory School (Mayhew and Edwards, 1936) and Jane Addams' (1925) Hull House were two examples of community outreach efforts based on pragmatic principles ('Tribute to Eleanor Clarke Slagle,' 1938, p. 13). In addition, the Arts and Crafts Society, housed at Hull House, was founded in Chicago by Professor Oscar Triggs (1902), another University colleague.

Hull House was a center where philosophy and practicality met. Julia Lathrop and Dewey conducted a club there devoted to the study of philosophy (Addams, 1935), and the center was used to meet the social and health needs of the community. The University and the Hull House community formed a tight network of scholars and practitioners devoted to pragmatism and its demonstration. Their focus was on meeting the needs of the individual and the needs of society in mutual benefit, an idea inherent in the philosophy of pragmatism. Hull House was a center where the themes of pragmatism were tried in the community in many forms. One such experiment was the CSCP (Addams, 1935).

Pragmatism as a philosophy is based on developmental and relational theories of Darwin and Hegel (Ayer, 1968). It describes the growth of knowledge through change and adaptation. It is a concept of holism, where the parts and the whole and the relationship between them are substantiated. It is a philosophy of mind/body integration and time/space unity. Pragmatism is considered a philosophy of time, history, or evolution because of its concern with the relationship or continuity between aspects of change. These concepts of time and evolution are addressed by Meyer (1922) and by Emil G. Hirsch (1892). The latter was a founder of the University of Chicago (D.E. Hirsch, 1968) and of CSCP (Dunton, 1915). Pragmatism assumes that change is adaptive, that human development and function recapitulate phylogenetic and historical sequences, and that active participation contributes to the development of the individual and society as a whole. Pragmatism describes the development of knowledge of the world for the individual and for society. This knowledge development progresses through egocentric, exocentric and consensual orientations (Breines, 1986a, 1986b). Therefore, reality is seen as ever changing, and it is evaluated through the relationships between the self and the concrete world of structure and society. The development of the individual proceeds throughout life, through active experience in that world, and from feedback provided by that experience. Pragmatism was adopted as a model for learning by Dewey, and as a model for health and social welfare by the mental hygienists, including Lathrop, Addams, Slagle, Meyer, and Hirsch (Cohen, 1983; Slagle, c. 1917).

The mental hygienists believed that these concepts of development and flux could be used to build health (Cohen, 1983). Health through active occupation, a principle of the mental hygiene movement, was the principle that guided the founders of the first school and early practitioners of occupational therapy in their applications in many areas of health care. However, of the founders of the profession, only Susan Tracy (1918) made Dewey's premises explicit for occupational therapy, and only she (Barrows, 1917) and George Barton (1914) verbalized active occupation's social themes and implications for health. The others demonstrated them.

Active occupation as a modifier of learning and health, a theme of great social relevance in the early part of the century (Dewey, 1916), received less emphasis as time went by. Instead, occupational therapists focused on their tools (Mosey, 1981).

The principles underlying occupation as they were defined by the founders of the profession, must be taught to students. The profession needs to become aware that newer theories can be compatible with the profession's original thinking. We must make the following clear:

1. Time and space, mind and body are unified in active occupation.
2. Active occupation structures development for the individual and for society.
3. Human development progresses from orientations of egocentricity to exocentricity and consensuality, replicating evolution.
4. All elements of performance influence one another because of the interactive nature of all systems.
5. The subjective nature of human beings is reflected in their performance and must be respected.
6. The uniqueness of individuals is counter-balanced by their relationship with their community.
7. Science and philosophy must be united to understand and enhance human occupation.
8. Grading activity along evolutional and developmental sequences enhances learning and performance, and therefore health.

These ideas which formed the basis for the founders' beliefs about occupational therapy are themes inherent in the philosophy of pragmatism. If these themes are made explicitly, students learning to be occupational therapists can recognize the purpose and relationships of the material they must study, despite the diversity of the topics. Neglecting to make explicit the relationship between our foundational philosophy and our educational system inhibits the synthesis for the student, for only some students are capable of creating this synthesis on their own. This fragmenting effect is antithetical to the principles of occupational therapy and the precepts of pragmatism. Seeing the wholes and the parts and their relationships to one another is vital if one is to understand human performance.

In my recent book, (Breines, 1986b) I developed a schematic for the structure of educational programs, which takes into account the overall concept of the profession, as well as the component aspects of individual curricula and institutions. The schematic represents an approximation of the topics that ordinarily compose the education of occupational therapists, organized according to a developmental systems approach. It is meant to expose the varied focus of occupational therapy education. However, it should be noted that this fractioning is artificial; no experience can separate the egocentric, exocentric, and consensual aspects of life's activities. Table 1.1 represents this model for curriculum design. If occupation therapy curricula are built on this model, faculty members and students will be able to recognize the relationship and relevance of the diverse course content to the conceptual whole of the curriculum.

It is acknowledged that, for many reasons, courses at different schools differ in content, sequence, and emphasis. Additionally, students come to occupational therapy education with greatly varying skills and preparation. Despite this diversity of education and preparation, I propose that the model presented here can provide a common structure on which communication can be built and a synthesis can be effected. The model is designed to serve as an example for the analysis of specific educational curricula. It can provide the wherewithal for assessing the content of individual curricula and can serve as an example for particularizing models of individual curricula so that they can be used as teaching tools for integrated learning. With such a structure, change can continue, permitting a constant upgrading of course content, while retaining and making explicit the conceptual framework to which the profession's founders adhered.

Table 1.1 A conceptual organization of occupational therapy curricula

	Subsubconcepts	*Subconcepts*	*Egocentricity*	*Exocentricity*	*Consensuality*
General topics	Physics Chemistry	Biology Neurology Medicine	Kinesiology Perception Learning theory Anatomy Psychology Sexuality	Crafts Sports Cooking Computers	Group theory Group therapy Sociology Anthropology Sexuality Parenting Vocations Communications
Occupational Therapy topics		Graded activities Activity analysis Activity synthesis	NDT PNF Sensory stimulation Body image, scheme Gnosis	SI Stereognosis ADL Adaptive equipment Splinting	Play/Leisure Augmentative communication Task groups Prevocational training Vocational roles

Notes: NDT = neurodevelopmental treatment; PNF = proprioceptive neuromuscular facilitation; SI = sensory integration; ADL = activities of daily living.

Source: From Origins and Adaptations: A Philosophy of Practice (p. 281) by E. Breines, 1986, Lebanon, NJ: Geri-Rehab. Copyright 1986 by E. Breines. Reprinted by permission.

Thinking Deep Thoughts

Occupational therapy is both simple and complex, concurrently. People who are receiving therapy are often engaged in simple, sometimes mundane, activities such as self care, crafts, games, or other ordinary occupations. In fact, the activities of practice are usually so simple from the perspective of the general public that occupational therapy practice itself seems ordinary, which affects our image. Haven't we had to live with the appellation of basket weaver, used as a metaphor for denigrating our practice?

However, simple activities are only simple if one can do them easily. They are not simple for persons with disabilities.

Most of the activities we do every day were learned when we were children. Few of us even remember when we learned how to do them. We hold a pencil and write, use a toothbrush and even drive a car without thinking about how we do that. By the time we became skilful at any task, they have become so simple that we tend no longer to hold them in high regard. After all, everyone can do them.

So here we are, skilled practitioners, teaching patients how to do simple things that the world, and even we, thinks are simplistic. What a dilemma for the practitioner who works in a sophisticated world of health care among other practitioners who speak in a language that seems mysterious, anything but simple, to the general public. It is difficult to ignore the comparison.

In actuality, occupational therapy derives from sophisticated thinking that is philosophical at origin. Understanding occupational therapy requires a more sophisticated approach than is readily apparent when one observes a patient in a practice environment.

Beyond the uncertainty often experienced by patients asked to do difficult tasks that were formerly easy, and the disparity between the principles held by other health providers and our own, there is a disconnection between our own view of activity as simple and our recognition of occupational therapy's complexity. Just envision, for example, the complexity of activity analysis. Books and articles have been written about this extensively examined topic.

This chapter includes a number of articles that attempt to bridge the gap between the simplicity and the complexity of occupational therapy by integrating philosophical notions with everyday practice. Some of the topics that appear in these articles include: purposefulness, evolution and adaptation, pragmatism, automatic and deliberate behavior, aesthetics, culture and semiotics.

Draw from these notions what you will. It is hoped they will encourage you to think about our profession in new ways that will enhance your ability to share sophisticated notions with your colleagues and, at the same time, enhance your pride in what we do and how we do it as health providers.

Occupational genesis: how activity, individual connect

Originally published in *Advance for Occupational Therapy* Dec. 18, 1995

Purposeful activity and occupation are at the core of our profession's history and philosophy. However, many therapists today have a limited understanding of these topics. Judging by the recent extended and enlightening discussion on Occu-list Serve, an electronic chat room emanating from Canada, scholars and educators are still seeking to better understand these fundamental concepts and find better ways to teach them.

My own dissertation research in 1986 identified occupational therapy's foundations in the philosophy of pragmatism and its historical proponents, John Dewey, William James, Rabbi Emil Hirsch, Adolf Meyer, Jane Addams and Julia Lathrop. (All of them knew Eleanor Clarke Slagle.)

Pragmatism, expressed in part by Dewey as 'learning by doing', is based on a historical and developmental model. It is sensitive to the evolutional theory of Darwin, and its theme of adaptation, which occupational therapy adopted, is built on the principle later advanced by systems theory.

All things influence one another in pragmatism's relational phenomenon. Through these influences, the individual contributes to society, and society contributes to the individual. These beliefs were promoted by Meyer, Slagle, Hirsch, Addams, Lathrop and James, who were members of the Mental Hygiene Society, and occupational therapists adopted the beliefs; but the core concepts of this philosophy have never been well understood by therapists.

Three essential components influence one another in 'active occupation', the term that Dewey advanced in 1916, a year prior to the founding of the National Society for the Promotion of Occupational Therapy – forerunner of the American Occupational Therapy Association.

The three essentials are:

- the individual, expressed in terms of mind and body;
- the tangible features of the world, expressed in terms of time and space;
- and the social environment, expressed in terms of language, culture, family and other social groups.

I have come to call the phenomena that result from this equation 'occupational genesis'.

Using this approach, one can analyze historically activities in which people have engaged from earliest times to the present, understanding them in their cultural meaningfulness. Similarly, activity also can be analyzed developmentally, and its meaningfulness dictated accordingly.

When an activity is vital to one's survival, it naturally has greater meaning than when it is viewed as non-essential or irrelevant. Within any given group, the more people who recognize the value of an activity, the more value it will have within that group.

At the same time, activities can be meaningful to individuals without being survival-related.

And so we as a profession have a dilemma, particularly in the United States. We live in a society in flux, composed of people of vastly different backgrounds, educational and economic levels, with values and interests that differ widely.

We ply our trade within educational and medical culture systems that hold different beliefs from our own. Our elders are attempting to teach our youngsters the old values, while the systems in which we work are changing beyond the experience of those elders.

How do we meet these varying needs? The pragmatists would say that meeting human needs requires sensitivity to individuals and their cultures.

It is a longstanding belief of occupational therapists that the patient/client should direct therapy. In order for the therapist to facilitate this, his or her own personal preferences must necessarily be subordinated to those of the patient. If activity is our essential tool, then it is vital that we learn as many activities as possible so we can use them as tools when they are appropriate.

Crafts are one of those tools. So are computers. So are self-care techniques. Very few therapists use all their tools all the time, but they are prepared through their education to be able to use them when necessary.

This column was designed to add some skills to the repertoire of therapists, so that when they are called upon, they have some resources upon which to draw.

There are profound ideas that underlie our practice. So I would advise, in terms of occupational therapy tools: don't throw the baby out with the bathwater because you personally can't find a rationale for its use. Instead, arm yourself with a fuller understanding of the beliefs that were instrumental to the founding of the profession, and how they were historically applied in terms of treatment.

If you do this, you will acquire greater confidence in your skills through reliance upon tools of your own choice. And you will be better prepared to articulate your work to others.

What do you know about spatial orientation?

Originally published in *Advance for Occupational Therapy* June 14, 1999

It's been some time since I had to move. I have lived in a wonderful house on a small farm in western New Jersey for the past 25 years. If I am lucky I don't anticipate having to move from there soon, if ever. But recently I accepted a new position at Seton Hall University, and I had to move my stuff.

I cannot remember ever feeling so disoriented. The disruption attached to having moved my files and my books left me with night terrors. In which box had I put which book? Where were all the boxes? Where were my notes about 'work hardening' and 'aging'? Where had I filed my handouts on occupational therapy theory and activity analysis? It seemed as if all my ring binders looked alike. Most were black, three inches wide, and had the labels falling off. It hadn't mattered that the labels were loose when I could reach up and find the binders exactly where I knew they were on the shelf. But moving them had dislodged the labels; and now the binders were in boxes, and the boxes were under or on top of other boxes, and I felt so lost.

I am usually a reasonably intact person, with an average sort of memory, albeit with some senior moments. Yet, this disruption was extraordinarily disturbing. How must people with extreme assaults to their psyches caused by physical or mental disability feel as a result of the disruptions they have in their life spaces?

Too often we forget that the patients we see in treatment environments are suffering as much from disruptions in spatial orientation as they are from their disabilities. Every patient who is admitted to a hospital or residential health care facility must experience this phenomenon. Making one's space one's own is as vital to recovery as is the attention that is being paid to the disability. We learn about space by establishing internalized coordinates based on the relationships between vertical, horizontal and depth. We begin that process early in development, probably in utero, and continue it throughout life each time we actively encounter new environments.

The inner ear is an active organ that governs our knowledge of space. However, activity is a vital element in the establishment of that knowledge. When one is ill, these important organs that organize one's perception of space are not stimulated, and one's sense of space is diminished through inactivity.

Likewise, the movement activity engenders is orienting. Activity that elicits and reinforces the development of spatial organization can enhance one's ability to perform activity in space. So it appears that activity enhances spatial orientation, and enhanced spatial orientation facilitates one's ability to perform activity.

It is important for us to recognize the various aspects of activity that contribute to spatial orientation, so that we can incorporate this knowledge into our treatment of patients. As experts in activity analysis, we are fully capable of making a fuller analysis of the orientational aspects of performance in order to structure treatment more effectively.

Clinical procedures can contribute to or diminish spatial awareness. It can be very disorienting to patients who are bedridden if others move them from place to place. One of the best ways for these patients to become better oriented is to move on their own in short excursions from and to their own rooms and beds. Learning wheelchair skills may be fundamental to the development of skill in other performances, as it aids orientation.

The health care community recognizes that mobility contributes to general healthfulness, but rarely notes that self-induced movement within space leads to increased orientation to that space. Yet, that is the basis of the theory of cognitive mapping. Studies indicate that for children, cognitive mapping is both a neurological and acquired developmental process. However, for adults, the recapitulation of that process has been less apparent, especially for those who have become disabled. The relationship between activity and spatial orientation should be more fully explored. Undoubtedly, there are many ways people define their spaces.

As for me, I am now re-organizing. I am sorting my ring binders. I am making new labels, putting my books into categories, and I am finding logical places to store my stuff at home and at work. And I am feeling much better now, thank you.

The end of occupational therapy? We have a choice

Originally published in *Advance for Occupational Therapy* May 3, 1999

Last week I saw an occupational therapist working with a patient, and I feared for my profession. It was not that what she was doing was so terrible, but rather what she was not doing.

I saw her put wrist weights on the patient and direct him to raise his hands while holding a cane, for a prescribed number of lifts. I saw her hook him up to a set of pulleys secured to the ceiling and set him to moving them back and forth.

There was no question that his arms would need to be strong so he could recover from his knee replacement, but these were the wrong muscles she was addressing, and more importantly, this patient lives in a two-story house, where his bedroom and bath are upstairs and the kitchen downstairs. The dogs he raises also live downstairs. Yet not one word was said about this dilemma and the implications his lifestyle and his disability had for each other.

How do I know this? The patient is a friend of mine. Strangely, when my friend introduced me as an occupational therapy educator, the therapist told me she thought she had not received a good education at the occupational therapy school she had attended. I didn't ask which she viewed as the school's shortfall: insufficient instruction on reductionistic treatment techniques or too much of the same.

The event disturbed me greatly, and I wasn't sure exactly why until I started reading Edward Wilson's book *Consilience*, in which he brilliantly merges concepts of philosophy, science and art in a comprehensive study of the evolution of humanity and the implications of this evolution on the future of humanity.

In the past few years, I have observed occupational therapists' delivery of services respond to pressures to become increasingly standardized and mechanistic. In some environments it has become so ritualized that I almost think anyone could do it! And as a matter of fact, other professions have come to assume that, indeed, they can, and they are attempting to do so. With the advent of restrictive funding, the squeeze is on. Everyone is compelled to move faster, deliver less, and compete, compete, compete! There seems to be a never-ending reduction of services, to be delivered, in the end, by anyone who can be trained to put on the weights to lift the cane, or pull the pulleys. Soon, no professional need be paid to perform these stylized tasks.

We can continue with this clear direction toward our destruction as a profession, as we do when we follow standardized pathways in treatment and education, or we can choose another path.

Occupational therapy is built on brilliant concepts of philosophy, science and art, merged in a comprehensive form that leads to the solution of problems. Darwin's concepts of evolutional and adaptation, Dewey's recognition of the value of 'learning through doing' and his comprehensive understanding of the integration of mind and body with time, space and social influences ground our thinking. These are the essential aspects of human occupation on living performance.

This information is delivered to occupational therapy students when they learn how human beings, with their minds and bodies, respond to their tangible and social environments in the performance of activities of all sorts. This is exactly what happens when students learn how to do activities with a variety of media and tools. The background and training of occupational therapists in activities that were/are important to the survival of ancient and modern peoples provides them with the skills they need to teach patients to be adaptive in their many and unique environments as the world changes around them in unanticipated ways.

Life's tasks can never be reduced to standardized, mechanistic methods of performance. Individuals are unique. Each has a set of skills and traits and lives in a personal environment that requires uniquely adaptive interaction. At the same time, that individual is involved in a unique culture and set of interactive relationships with family and society.

These variables are too many to be reduced to pro forma procedures. The occupational therapist's unique skill is recognizing and manipulating the variables to assist the person in reaching life goals. Every experienced therapist knows it is fruitless to provide the same set of adaptive tools to patients with the same diagnosis. These are the things the home care therapist finds in the closet or used for purposes the therapist never dreamed of, often by family members who did not receive the items at the outset.

So here is our choice. We can follow the road to extinction by eliminating what appear to be unscientific skills, or we can value and emulate the paths taken by our predecessors. When we learn activities, we do not learn them only to teach them to patients. We learn them so that we become competent in the use and analysis of all the potential tools and materials around us, and understand their relevance and meaning to people, so that we can use them in adaptive ways when the time comes.

The health care system as we have known it is imploding around us as society attempts to achieve cost savings. Yet using reductionistic methods in rehabilitation is shortsighted and limiting. Discharging patients from treatment before they have reached their maximum capacity for recovery leaves all of us with greater costs over the long run. Human problems can be solved only by understanding and interacting with human beings in their entire capacity. That's what we do best.

Personally, I opt for survival. What's your choice?

Never mind who we are – what do we do?

Originally published in *Advance for Occupational Therapy* Jan. 25, 1999

We used to argue about what we called ourselves. We went from reconstruction aides to occupational therapists. Even now we have used or heard the terms 'functional therapist', 'activity therapist', 'hand therapist', 'developmental therapist', 'psych therapist' and others used to refer to us. But the most recent debate seems to be centered on what to call what we do. Are we providing occupation as treatment? Or is it purposeful activity we use?

More and more I read arguments that say we should delete the word 'activities' from our lexicon and substitute the word 'occupation'. No more activity analysis. Now it is to be occupational task analysis. The first time I heard it suggested that we delete the word 'activity' from our vocabulary was when Dr David Nelson presented his Eleanor Clarke Slagle Lecture several years ago at national conference. His students got up and displayed their T-shirts, which had printed on them the word 'activity' in a circle with a line through it just like traffic signs forbidding U turns. A number of individuals have taken up the cause and begun to promulgate this idea.

That we should delete the word 'activity' seemed like a logical argument when I first heard it. I nearly renamed the title of this column! But I thought about it for a while and began to have some reservations. Deleting from practice and literature a word that represents what occupational therapists have been doing for so long seems somewhat risky in the long term.

I remember when Gail Fidler warned the profession in the early 1970s that it was giving up too much when it delivered a whole aspect of what we had traditionally incorporated in our practice to others. Dance therapists. Art therapists. Recreation therapists. Horticulture therapists, etc. Prior to that time, occupational therapists used all of these media in their practice realm. Many still do. The issue at the time hung on the fact that occupational therapists wanted to be perceived as more scientific and at the same time receive fee-for-services rendered rather than provide services to institutions as a whole in which charges were reflected in day rates. So occupational therapists moved away from their identity in activities and closer to the medical science arena. Is it any wonder that occupation therapy practice began to look less activity-based?

Now, occupational therapists have begun once again to value occupation and promote our identity within its definitions. This is a good thing. It should be welcomed. Yet at the same time they reject an identity that uses the term activity. My feeling is that unless occupational therapists learn to value activity as a dimension of occupation, they will not overcome their uncertainty about their professional identity.

We must develop pride in what we do. Hiding our identity under a word deletion is not a healthy way to develop that pride. There is no shame in using activities for their therapeutic effect. The activities do not become more meaningful because they are called occupations. And if our understanding of occupations is to exclude aspects of activity, we are back to eliminating aspects of practice that have proven to be healthful. Again we will be giving away our expertise by doing so.

And as Mary Reilly stated, someone will certainly enter the void to take up our role.

It seems to me that we often are our own worst enemies. Instead of instilling pride in our students and colleagues, we too often encourage inadequacy. Our politics should not be such that we promote only words we think are to our advantage, but rather that we alter first our own feelings about our roles and how we describe them. And that we then promote ourselves within that identity.

Purposeful activities have a long and valuable heritage for the profession, and for a significant philosophy upon which the profession was built. John Dewey, the philosopher of pragmatism and education, spoke of active occupation and purposive activity in 1916, one year before the founding of the National Society for the Promotion of Occupational Therapy (which became the American Occupational Therapy Association). His recognition of the importance of purpose in activity and occupation, and the use of both terms may be telling. Let's not throw out the baby with the bath water. Before we advocate for the use of one of these terms to the detriment of the other, let's recognize that there is value in both. It is never a problem when we have more ways to express ourselves.

It's what you don't have to think about that counts

Originally published in *Advance for Occupational Therapy* Aug. 19, 1996

One of my favorite quotations is by Alfred North Whitehead, the famous philosopher:

> *It is a profoundly erroneous truism, repeated by all copy books, and by eminent people when they are making speeches, that we should cultivate the habit of thinking what we are doing. The precise opposite is the case. Civilization advances by extending the number of important operations we can perform without thinking about them.*

The reason this quotation intrigues me so is that I think it makes a great case for our use of active occupation as a therapeutic tool.

Whitehead is correct that most individuals think it is important to pay attention to what we are doing. We can all remember being admonished by our teachers, our parents, our coaches to 'pay attention'. And try as we might, paying attention didn't seem to be the answer. We made mistakes no matter how hard we concentrated. The problem was, we were only able to pay attention to one thing at a time.

Clean your room, forget your homework. Hold the racket high, and lose your footing. It seemed that if one thing was right, something else went wrong. And the problem was always, 'You weren't paying attention.'

But what if paying attention is the wrong premise? Maybe we should not be paying attention. Maybe we should be disregarding.

What a novel idea! Being able to perform without paying attention may be exactly what we should be about.

Quite remarkably, that is precisely what occupational therapists are largely intent on, and have been since the profession was founded. From the beginning, the concept of habit training has been a strong component of practice. Eleanor Clarke Slagle knew that habits could be developed, and her therapy program focused on this aspect. With good habits, performance could be positively structured, enhancing patients' ability to function in their life skills.

To encourage good habits, she developed a program of well integrated occupational tasks that included active occupation, rest and play. Self care, farming, handcrafts, industrial occupations, games and exercise were offered in measured quotients, contributing to the development of a healthy lifestyle.

Along with these concepts came an understanding of 'goal (or task) oriented'. Essentially, this term came to represent the idea that one performed some aspects of tasks automatically and some deliberately. That is, the end goal was in conscious attention, but in order to achieve the end goal, one had to perform other aspects of the task automatically.

So, as one reached to make the weaving grow, the trunk shifted and compensated to allow the task to be performed. Attention was not to the trunk, or even to the grasp but instead was to the weaving itself. The leather lacing required grasp, reach, perceptual organization, strength – but the stitch was the object under examination. If it was correctly done, the performance was apparent.

And even if incorrect, the strength and dexterity had been engaged, albeit outside of conscious attention.

Joy Huss described the implications of this idea for therapy as follows: 'You can spend hours teaching Johnny to hold his head up or straighten his elbow voluntarily. He can learn to do it consciously. But if you give him anything else to think about at the same time, he will not be able to hold his head up or reach for an object.'

It appears that some things can be done consciously only one at a time. In order for aspects of activity to be performed in concert, some have to be done without attention. As a matter of fact, that is the purpose of reflexes. Nature has provided us with some skills the potential for which are delivered at birth.

Nursing babies turn to the breast because nature has endowed them with the capacity to do so. They can concentrate on getting the milk because they do not have to concentrate on how to find it. Babies learn to stack blocks because their ability to grasp and release enables them to concentrate on the blocks. Children can run only when they can walk without think about it. They can play running games only when they can run without concentrating on their feet.

Throughout life, the ability to gain skills is dependent on being able to perform subskills automatically. One is considered proficient only when one can perform the essential aspects of a task without concentrating on them. Being able to perform automatically is inherently safe. If one were unable to drive without concentrating on the brake, the gas pedal, or the turn signal, few of us would leave the driveway.

So remember, if I can paraphrase Whitehead, our patients advance by extending the number of important operations they can perform without thinking about them. And the key to that performance is the diversion that active occupations provide.

The thinker and the sower

Originally published in *Advance for Occupational Therapy* July 13, 1998

I suppose it started when I saw Rodin's stunning sculptures of 'The Thinker' and 'The Sower'.

I had just arrived in Quebec City from Montreal, where I was attending the Congress of the World Federation of Occupational Therapists, and the Rodin pieces were on exhibit there.

I was struck with the intense unity of mind and body exemplified by 'The Thinker' who seems almost intensely in pain. What was he thinking about, bent forward with his head on his hand?

Still wondering, I glanced at the 'The Sower'. This active sculpture shows a man vigorously at work, preparing his fields. His face looks forward and exhibits hope and satisfaction.

Is Rodin confiming to us through his artistry that thinking without action may be less healthful than occupation that generated satisfactory ends – the harvest, for example?

Perhaps more important is that this one artist's metaphors were more crystallizing and enlightening for me than so many thought-provoking lessons about my own profession.

At WFOT, I noticed, international boundaries are not restrictive of thinking or doing for occupational therapists. While the words we use to describe ourselves and what we do may differ, as demonstrated by Nelson and Johannsen's study of the international languages and meaning of occupation, the underlying beliefs about what we represent seem more similar than different. Active doing in meaningful occupation permeates our belief systems.

But I found that knowing explicitly how to use activity as therapy seems more dependent on cultural and legal issues related to political economics. Attendance at the conference seemed to be more readily supported by member countries with social welfare systems than by nations who are restricted by the economics of reimbursement funding.

As I moved from session to session, trying to soak up as much information as I could in the brief few days I was in Montreal, I found myself choosing carefully among the many presentations. I found that many of the poster sessions were exciting. In fact, they gave me more flexibility in time and choices. I could dwell on the posters I found interesting, and walk quickly by those that did not catch my interest. If the posters were crowded, one could always return, and the opportunity to speak with the presenters was more available than in the presentations, which were strictly limited by time.

As a poster presenter myself, I found it very interesting to speak with people from around the world about my own work. Never mind that standing most of the day was hurting my feet. Here mind and body spoke loudly to one another.

Oddly enough, I kept bumping into the same people over and over in the various sessions I selected. As activity analysis is a perpetual activity of mine, I began to apply this to the topics I was pursuing, analyzing them for their content. I found no surprise there. It seems that I was gravitating to topics that were philosophical, spiritual and analytical. Presentations about Taoism, ritual and creativity intrigued me. How surprised I was to find many of the same people gravitating to these same topics. Now I know which of my colleagues appreciate dialogue about these esoteric but vital concepts.

Most fun of all were the little notes that were posted on the message boards informing people of mutual interests and opportunities. For example, 'Meet at 4 p.m. to learn origami.' And meet we did. On the floor of the upper lobby, folding our little colored pieces of paper while getting to know people from all the continents of the world.

The international flavor of the event was evident in the various costumes, the alternative spellings and alphabets, and the many sounds of language. Unfamiliar accents required careful attending.

All this just added to the excitement, if not to sensory overload. It struck me that in doing, human beings usually make evident their intent while they struggle with the weight of resistance, the problems of living, and others who are dependent on the activity. Their bodies reveal their intensity of thought.

And I am sure I would not have seen a message in 'The Thinker' and 'The Sower' if I had not been properly prepared by merging my mind and body in my own meaningful activity.

Consider cultural influences when teaching patients activities of daily living

Originally published in *Advance for Occupational Therapy* April 21, 1997

One of the most important terms in the language of our profession is 'activities of daily living'. Yet we rarely thing of ADL when we think about activities. Perhaps it's time to analyze these ADL just as we do other forms of activity.

This issue came up in our Introduction to Occupational Therapy class the other day when we were discussing the need to understand the influence of culture on patients' behaviors. We began to think about the many aspects of culture that are part of our understanding of ADL. We are fortunate that our classes are generally representative of diverse cultural groups, and the faculty encourages students to treat classes as cultural laboratories so they can learn about customs from each other. Once the students get to know one another, they are generally eager to share their traditions and customs.

One of our students is from the island of Jamaica. She told us that when she came to the United States, she was surprised to find that the women shave their legs. Similarly, some of the American-born students told us how shocked they were when they visited European countries and found that not only did the women not shave their legs, but their bathing rituals and time frames were completely different.

In Europe, it is generally not expected that one bathe every day, and it is certainly not considered necessary to wash one's hair daily. In class, we talked some about plumbing, fresh water, fuel supplies and the economy, and the class began to understand why people would have different bathing practices and expectations.

So as not to exclude men in the class, I asked one young man about the length of his beard. He said he sported a beard because he was lazy and didn't want to be bothered shaving every day in the week. The short beard that I observed each week was because that's how long it gets by Tuesday when our class meets. I asked him how he would feel if a therapist came in and said, 'It's time to shave.' He said he would respond, 'Go right ahead.' But he surely had no intention of participating.

Then I turned to a young Orthodox rabbi in our class who sports a full beard. I said, 'What should we know about your beard and how you keep it in shape?' Although he did not shave, he described the special rules about cutting a beard that many Orthodox Jewish men follow. Based on biblical interpretations, only certain kinds of cutting implements are allowed for shaving.

At that point, one of the women in the class asked, 'What do I do when a patient of mine is Orthodox, has a beard, and is aphasic? How can I be sure I respect his cultural and religious practices?' The students were quick to realize that families are an excellent source, not only of ideas, but implements as well. Familiar tools from home that one is permitted to use can be brought into the clinic to use.

What stemmed from this discussion was a clear recognition that one's cultural identity strongly influences one's attitude and practices, even in the most intimate aspects of ADL. Those of us who live and work in New York City, where there are many first generation residents and people who live according to traditional rituals, see many people who wear a wide variety of clothing, from turbans, wigs, long skirts and wraps, to tight jeans and various fashion statements. Each of them have their own history. Some people observe religious rules that prohibit the wearing of some kinds of clothes. Still others are mandated to wear specific kinds of garb. There are even proscriptions against some kinds of fabrics and closures.

Toileting practices also differ from culture to culture. In some, the right hand is reserved for eating and the left for personal care. It is customary in some European countries for the toilet to be in one room, the water closet, while a separate room is reserved for the bath. The problems of toilet transfers differ in these environments. The use of a bidet is common in Europe, whereas it is uncommon in the United States. Some people are more apt to take a bath, whereas a shower is customary in the States. Each of these practices have their own particulars: washcloths or not, liquid or bar soaps, towels or sheets, etc.

Becoming familiar with different personal practices you are apt to encounter is a necessity if you are to be effective in teaching your patients ADL. These ideas are imbedded in their belief systems from childhood. If you do not take the time to learn about their familiar practices and the foundations of these practices, you are doomed to fail.

Activities of daily living are the most intimate and personal activities in which one engages. They were learned in early childhood and practiced throughout life. Imposing new methods of performing ADL on patients, without appreciating the techniques and customs that construct one's image of these activities has the possibility of violating long held beliefs. On the other hand, showing patients that you are respectful of their practices is more apt to enable you and your patients to succeed.

The origin of adaptation

Originally published in *Advance for Occupational Therapy* Jan. 19, 1998

One of the most interesting aspects of occupational therapy education is how it prepares us with abilities we need to adapt various activities to the needs of many different individuals, who are engaged in the activities. As a matter of fact, the most fundamental skill an occupational therapist has is analysis of activity.

This attention to our foundational skill comes early in the curriculum and is honed throughout our education, preparing us for its application in the clinical environment. The skill is further honed with experience.

Master clinicians demonstrate this ability masterfully. Yet few therapists recognize its source. The techniques are studied as technical skills, without much attention, if any, to the origin of the ideas which structure our abilities.

The concept of adaptation derives from the ideas presented in Charles Darwin's famous book, *The Origin of the Species by Means of Natural Selection*. Darwin believed that the environment structured the evolution of species, in that those that adapted to the environments in which they lived, survived, and those that were unable to adapt succumbed. Of these, we have only a fossil record.

Philosopher John Dewey adopted the premises of evolution in his theory of pragmatism and its application to education. Translating the evolutional model of phylogenetic origin to a developmental model of ontogenetic origin, Dewey recognized the integration of mind and body in the manipulation of environment led to learning based on constant curiosity fed by success.

The meaningful environment provides the just-right stimulus for this process. Thus his premise of learning through doing, a concept later adopted by occupational therapists.

Following the lead of the mental hygienists who were influenced by Dewey, occupational therapists carried this concept still further, applying the ideas to health as well as education. Successful adaptation was viewed not only as a natural phenomenon, but as one that could by stimulated by skilled clinicians. The environment could be adapted to enable the patient to perform successfully. Or, the patient could adapt so as to be able to perform.

Hence we had to learn to analyze activity. It is through this skill that we become able to determine whether to adapt the patient to the environment or the environment to the patient. The choices are only available when one can analyze the endless possibilities an activity provides.

Each activity in which we engage is constructed of a relationship between egocentric (mind-body), exocentric (time-space) and consensual qualities that are distinctive in their arrangement. Dusting the furniture has remarkably different qualities than does cycling. Digging a garden is different from knitting a sweater. Each activity makes different demands on the mind and body, and requires different skills. Each activity is enabled by different skills. Each activity is enabled by different tools and equipment used in very specific ways.

And each meets the needs of society in a different way as the individual engaged in the activity participates in life roles. Understanding these various elements is vital to being able to adapt person or environment to those roles. Feather-duster or rag, 10-speed or tricycle, raised garden bed or modified space, coarse yarn or fine needles, are all choices one has available in the adaptation of activity.

Therapists must be able to perform a variety of activities in order to skillfully adapt them and understand their influence on people. Consequently, I believe that occupational therapists have a professional responsibility and a lifetime of work ahead of them in acquiring various skills.

Adapting activity is secondary to this understanding. It includes a whole other set of skills that incorporate a knowledge of human function in its normal and abnormal manifestations throughout the lifespan. Since all occupational therapists have these skills, we are perfectly well adapted to deliver practice based upon them.

Thank you Darwin, Dewey, James, Meyer, Hirsch, Lathrop and Slagle.

We need to talk the talk

Originally published in *Advance for Occupational Therapy* Feb. 11, 2002

We get so caught up today in what to call what we do. The term 'occupation' has overtaken our lexicon and every author expounds on it at length. On the other hand, the term 'activity' has taken a lesser place (even if it is in the title of this column). And still lower on the food chain is 'crafts'. That word is almost never used in the occupational therapy literature nowadays, even though the notion of satisfying and productive leisure time seems to be expanding in the public eye. It seems that if we call something 'occupation', we can lay claim to it; if we call it crafts, we shy away.

I have to wonder why we are so reluctant to use the terms crafts and activities, even though they represent ideas that are so familiar to the public. Is it because the use of homely words makes us think that we are demeaning ourselves?

I have written at some length about the idea that occupational therapy practitioners need to be proud of themselves before they can expect others to respect them. I believe that if we had genuine pride in the ideas and behaviors that represent our profession, we would be comfortable in using all forms of the language. I also believe that it may be a mistake to use stilted language to describe our work. Using unfamiliar language to describe what we do does not help to make our work more familiar and comfortable to other people.

So how would we go about moving ourselves forward so that we are comfortable with all the tools we use?

I wonder if just changing our language to be more inclusive would be effective in changing our attitudes.

I've noticed that our students today are much more willing to accept crafts as a therapeutic tool than are the students I used to have a few years ago. Is it that times have changed? Or is it that they are becoming more comfortable faster?

One of the techniques I use to accommodate students to crafts is to explain these activities in terms of the trades. We don't look at crafts as only diversional. We expose them as forms of work that people used to engage in to make a living, and in many instances still do today.

For example, ceramics is akin to masonry. Many of the same tools and materials are used. Carpentry and construction are other trades that use many of the same woodworking skills and tools we use in lab. Jewelers use them in metal crafts. Paper and printing activities are evident in many kinds of work people do.

Once students are able to see these activities as valuable in various aspects of people's lives, they seem to be able to accept them as basic tools for therapy. I am certain that the attitudes they develop towards crafts early in their occupational therapy education enables them to recognize their usefulness as therapeutic tools.

Needless to say, I am delighted when students come back from fieldwork and explain how they introduced the use of crafts and other activities into clinics where they were previously unused. And the feedback we get from the clinics is very positive as well.

I believe that the underutilization of crafts can be attributed in part to the era when occupation itself was virtually eliminated from occupational therapy curricula around the country in an attempt to make us more scientific. Some old timers like myself held on. Now I'm pleased to say that some youngsters are on board.

The next thing we need is some evidence for the worth of activities in enhancing health. It would be an awful shame if some other professional group would take credit for what occupational therapy has had mastery in from its inception. Once we can show that the work we do is effective in making positive changes, I think we'll have less difficulty in bragging about what we do.

And I'll bet we find that we will be more comfortable in using the language that reflects what we do, whether it is occupation, activity, crafts, trades, work or leisure.

Genesis of occupation: a philosophical model for therapy and theory

Originally published in *Australian Occupational Therapy Journal* March 1990, 37(1): 45–9

Abstract

Occupational genesis is an evolution/developmental theme based on concepts developed by the philosophers of pragmatism, Dewey, James, Mead and Pierce. Their influence on the Chicago community where occupational therapy originated is described.

By bringing this philosophy to light as occupational therapy's conceptual foundation, modern theorists and practitioners can be understood to be united in their beliefs despite differences in practice orientations. This concept of pragmatic origin, to which Adolf Meyer adhered, is proposed as occupational therapy's central theme. Occupational genesis describes the development of function through orientation of egocentricity, exocentricity and consensuality, a sequence repeated throughout life in the acquisition of skill. The relationship is described between inherited and acquired automatic behavior and purposeful activity, and their roles in adaptive development. The relevance of this conceptual system for the profession and for health care is suggested.

Occupational therapy is based on a concept of occupational development or genesis, a theme advanced by the philosophers of pragmatism who provided the profession's conceptual foundation (Breines, 1986c). Occupational genesis adheres to G. Stanley Hall's theory that 'ontogeny recapitulates phylogeny', an evolutional and developmental tenet of pragmatism advanced by Adolf Meyer (1952). The development of occupation proceeds sequentially from the synthesis of automatic performances (whether reflexes or habits) with deliberate actions, through purposeful activity in adaptive interaction with structural and social environments. The acquisition of skill is viewed as a developmental process, in much the same manner that general systems theory (von Bertalanffy, 1962) describes this process as a feedback phenomenon. This progressively acquisitional process extends throughout life and throughout lifetimes, as the world is encountered and knowledge is synthesized toward adaptive functioning. Development results from the relationship that occurs between individuals and their structural and social environments. This concept was instrumental to the foundation of the profession, and remains so today.

Remarkably, occupational therapy retained this consistent philosophy throughout its history, although it did not have the privilege of knowing that it had a philosophy, nor that its philosophy was explicitly defined by scholars of world renown (Breines, 1986c). Occupational therapists were given a great heritage by the individuals who taught the profession's founders, but the founders' neglect to make explicit the foundational concepts of the profession created problems in understanding. If the pragmatic concept of occupational genesis had been made explicit by the founders, one would suspect that feelings of inadequacy and questions of identity expressed throughout the profession's history would not have developed.

Yet these questions remain. Occupational therapists, for the most part, are uncertain as to their philosophical origins and continue to have difficulty explaining themselves to others (Hamer, 1984). That therapists are unable to clearly describe themselves to others, and even to themselves, results in feelings of inadequacy and frustration (Sachs, 1988). This paper proposes a framework for resolving these questions and the attendant feelings of inadequacy they engender by offering a comprehensive yet succinct concept that is relevant for all types of practice. With a concept easy for occupational therapists to understand, for it is clearly their belief system and with the knowledge that it comes out of a philosophy of recognized public acclaim, therapists can hold their heads high and articulate their identity with skill and sophistication. Furthermore, with such a philosophical foundation, it is anticipated that research and education will flourish in a manner that holds greater meaning for therapists as well as their colleagues and clients. For example, if problems that face the profession, such as new approaches to research methodology, questions of curriculum design and issues of professionalism (Breines, 1987, 1988a, 1988b) are viewed with an eye towards an explicit foundational philosophy in pragmatism, these problems may well be resolvable or moot.

An historical perspective on occupational therapy's view of its philosophy

Occupational therapy has been a formalized profession since it was established in 1917 at a meeting of its founders at Clifton Springs, New York. The first association of occupational therapists was called the National Society for the Promotion of Occupational Therapy (Licht, 1967; Hopkins and Smith, 1983; Colman, 1984). Despite their interest in promoting occupational therapy, the founders did not introduce an explicit philosophical rationale into the educational curriculum of the therapists (notes, c. 1918; Batchelder, 1985), leaving the impression in later years that occupational therapy was bereft of a philosophy (American Occupational Therapy Association, 1979a). A familiar but unsubstantiated theme offered to therapists was, 'We treat the whole person.' Activity analysis and grading of activities were the means by which this task was accomplished. But no conceptual framework was provided by which therapists could understand the unity of these principles and their relationship to a foundational philosophy. It was considered sufficient for the practitioner to be able to do the job.

This approach was satisfactory until the knowledge explosion of the modern era provided new techniques and rationales for practice based on scientific principles. Therapists began to have difficulty defining their practice. They could not explain neural treatment techniques, group process, vocational preparation, and arts and crafts in the same breath.

Out of this crisis, defined by Kielhofner (1982) in Kuhnian (1970) terms of paradigm shift, a number of models of occupation were put forth to explain the purpose of occupational therapy. These discussions took many directions and, while they were often unrelated or concurrent proposals, concern for a unifying concept appeared evident. Some of these concepts are described below.

Relying on White's (1963, 1971) efficacy concepts based on ego psychology theory, Fidler and Fidler (1978, 1981) described the value of purposeful activity in terms of the tangible evidence of competence it provided, determined in large part by responses from others. The value of therapy was viewed in terms of the emotional validation that was offered by seeing results of personal efforts, as well as by the feedback offered from the responses to those efforts by others. Llorens (1980), taking another approach, offered developmental theory as a foundation. Within this framework, she created a taxonomy in which elements she identified as performance components and occupational performances were described. With this approach, the organization she developed contributed a new perspective for the profession. Other conceptual organizations were also described. Among these, Kielhofner and Burke (1980) described human occupation. They built on Reilly's adherence to systems theory. Reilly (1974), in describing occupational behavior, presented systems theory as a means of understanding occupation. She emphasized play as a foundational component of human performance, during which preparation for subsequent social roles takes place. Each development and the acquisition of skill were viewed from a systems theory approach. Amplifying Reilly's perspective, Kielhofner and Burke described a hierarchy for components of performance, stipulating these as volition, habit and skill.

Still other therapists chose other theories upon which to structure their perspectives, However, the theories upon which occupational therapists built their models were insufficient in unifying a common conceptual organization. No resolution was made for the role of neural aspects of development in concert with systems theory and group concepts. Since each of these and other theories were valued by different and considerable segments of the profession, this evidence of splintering created a problem for describing an encompassing view of practice; several authors attempted to resolve this problem by making various well reasoned arguments toward synthesis (Lindquist, Mack, and Parham, 1982a, 1982b; Katz, 1985). However, their papers have been less than successful in resolving the discomfort felt by many practicing therapists. To see the concepts of Fidler, Reilly, and neurodevelopmental theorists such as Ayres (1972) in light of each other appears to have been beyond the ability or inclination of most therapists.

This difficulty was, and remains, heightened by the fact that therapists have been subject to the pressures of counter philosophies advanced by the facilities in which they were employed (Breines, 1986a, 1986c), in combination with their inability to articulate their own comprehensive philosophy. The emphasis on Cartesian scientific principles in health care institutions left little room for the subjective principles of the pragmatists in which many therapists are comfortable and skilled. For many, this division in values resulted in a split in identities, and raised questions for the profession, expressed partly as issues of specialization. As a result, therapists tended to identify with one or another scheme in order to resolve their conflict. They were supported in this fragmented approach by respected theorists such as Mosey (1970, 1985) who advanced 'frames of reference' and 'pluralism'. The voices who had cried out for a unified philosophy (Yerxa, 1979; AOTA, 1979a) were not silenced.

Pragmatism and its proponents

In the latter part of the nineteenth century, a concept was formulated which has been identified worldwide as the great American philosophy (Smith, 1978). It was a break from earlier conceptual forms, such as that exemplified by the thinking of Descartes whose statement, 'I think; therefore, I am', represents his view of the separation of mind and body (Mills, 1964). It is an attempt to clarify, by isolation, an approach inherent in much of scientific inquiry as practiced to date. This compartmentalized approach, the mind/body dichotomy of Descartes, was rejected by the pragmatists in favor of a belief in the unity of mind and body in action.

Four philosophers, Charles Peirce, John Dewey, William James and George Herbert Mead, are primarily identified with pragmatism (Ayer, 1968; Rorty, 1982). Together, they described a philosophy of history, holism and relationship. They concerned themselves with the influences of time and relationship on human activity. Time was the thread that ran through history and development, and was understood to influence knowledge and performance. The concepts of change and continuity were explored in depth. They argued that change occurs within the influence of prior events and therefore, past, present and future are inextricably connected. As a result, they understood change to be not a concept of compartmentalization but rather a concept of relationship or continuity. They applied these concepts to historical and phylogenetic events, as well as to developmental or ontogenetic events. In describing this extensive philosophy, other themes adopted by the pragmatists were doubt, habit, active occupation, 'purposive' activity (Dewey, 1916), transaction, and adaptation (Darwin, 1859).

The pragmatists believed that human action is structured by influences of the past, exemplified in part as inherited reflexes, and in part as learned habits. They believed that purposeful, adaptive, individual as well as communal experiences build on these less conscious performances and contribute to the growth and welfare of individuals and society. The pragmatists focused heavily on the subjectivity of experience, and the role of communion in discerning 'truth', amid the interrelated and myriad influences that time presents. They acknowledged that many threads of experience occur concurrently and consecutively. Furthermore, because of these many influences, individuals come to knowledge with unique perspectives. It was in communication and interaction between individuals that society grew, developed, and resolved the potential isolation of these unique perspectives. They understood these concepts in terms of the developing individual in a developing society. They adopted the subjective themes of relativity described by Einstein and Heisenberg, and underscored these themes as relevant for understanding human behavior (Mead, 1932). Human beings experience the world within a subjective reality, which becomes confirmed by feedback from the tangible and people world. It is within this potentially ambiguous environment that we grow and adapt.

The primary center for pragmatic study and the application of these ideas in social benefit was centered about the University of Chicago around the turn of the century. Those who belonged to this Chicago community included John Dewey, George Herbert Mead, Adolf Meyer and Mary Potter Brooks Meyer (Meyer, 1952), Rabbi Emil G. Hirsch (Dunton, 1915; Hirsch, 1968), Jane Addams (1925), Julia Lathrop (Addams, 1935), and Eleanor Clarke Slagle (Breines, 1986a), all of whom were important figures to the early development of the occupational therapy profession. They were friends and colleagues devoted to issues of social welfare, united in the their philosophical approach to the development of health and education (Cohen, 1983) through active occupation. They demonstrated in acts of social benefit that pragmatism was a philosophy of social as well as intellectual merit. The developmental concept to which they adhered in thinking and in action can be described as occupational genesis.

Occupational genesis

Occupational genesis describes a process of development of human performance which proceeds from an orientation that is egocentric (self oriented), to that which is exocentric (oriented to external objects and space), to that which is consensual (oriented to the beliefs or perspectives of others). Earliest performance is egocentered, and most structured by inherited features. Evolutional adaptation has assured for human beings certain capacities which have determined our survival. These egocentric capacities are normally most evident in earliest development, and are nature's protective mechanisms for survival. Subsequent performance is structured by these early parameters, yet develops in adaptation to a tangible environment, a phenomenon described here as exocentric. The influence of gravity and other forces are resolved as they interact with inherited capacities and purposeful activity, permitting a broadening of dimension spatial coordinates for performance. Active experience increases the knowledge of space and objects and enables adaptation to the environment. As performance matures, influences of a social nature become increasingly consensual, contributing to the adaptation of the individual to a developing society, in mutual interdependence.

None of these three elements of egocentricity, exocentricity and consensuality is to be interpreted as operating in isolation from one another; nor does an individual pass from one stage to another. All of these elements are present at all times throughout life, but they are biased to structure performance in a developmental order as the acquisition of new skills demands adaptive performance. Therefore, for each new acquisition, individuals are stimulated by doubt to solve life's problems, and their automaticity on one level enables further skill development at another level. For example, one must learn to move the body's parts in order to learn to manipulate tools, in order to be productive and contributing. Whether learning to suckle, to crawl, to ride a bicycle, or to operate a computer, one must recapitulate this egocentric, exocentric, consensual process of acquiring automation for each newly acquired skill.

An attempt has been made to reduce this concept to a graphic model in the hope that such visualization would contribute to the reader's understanding of the relationship between these elements. Figure 2 demonstrates the equivalent roles of phylogeny and ontogeny and the feedback that occurs between mind and body, as well as automaticity (reflex, habit, skill, subcortical) and deliberation (planning, purpose, will, cortical) in the development of functional performance in life span activities.

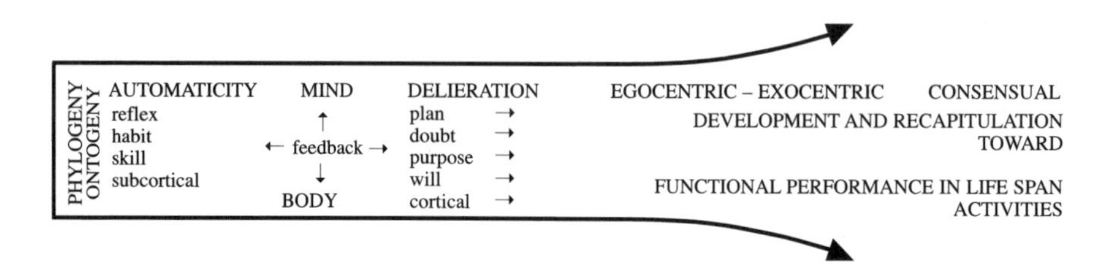

Figure 2: Model of occupational genesis.

Life is provocative and demands solution, whether one considers the problems of the individual or problems of society, infant or adult. The process is the same. As Alfred North Whitehead states:

> *It is a profoundly erroneous truism, repeated by all copy books, and by eminent people when they are making speeches, that we should cultivate the habit of thinking what we are doing. The precise opposite is the case. Civilization advances by extending the number of important operations we can perform without thinking about them. (Whitehead, 1957)*

The same is true for the individual. Therefore, continued development, whether of the individual or of society, is dependent upon automaticity. If you have to think about where or how to place your feet, you are unlikely to be able to find your destination, or even to imagine one.

When the concept of automaticity was introduced by the pragmatists, they united the concepts of phylogeny and ontogeny. Inherited automaticity (reflex) directs earliest experience. Acquired automaticity (habit and skill) enables later experience. Automaticity on either level is essential to purposeful activity. Purposeful activity can address only those components of performance for which underlying automatic behaviors exist, whether these are reflexes, habits or skills. Within this analysis, reflex does not have to be viewed as a mechanistic phenomenon. Rather, it is to be viewed as a phenomenon of automaticity, mirrored in human performance by habits or skills. It does not matter to performance whether the tasks we can perform automatically are inherited or acquired. It matters only whether those automatic elements of performance are adaptive, for the individual or for society. The pragmatists interpreted that, for the individual, these capacities are recapitulated in each generation; for the individual and for society, new dimensions build on the old.

Occupational therapists adapted this premise of development based on active experience, consistent with the pragmatist philosophical heritage they were given (albeit implicitly), and were comfortable with this theme. But they have been unable to explain it adequately, because they were uneducated about its influences, and they have suffered from the splintering and compartmentalizing influences of the Cartesian philosophy which underlies much of scientific inquiry and largely dictates the parameters of their workplaces. So they kept the elements of the pragmatists' philosophy, but delivered them in fragmented form. The paradigm shift in the profession referred to earlier was not so much a shift in belief systems, but rather, the author believes, a discomfiture expressed in an attempt to retain within practice the philosophical elements which had been described in the beginning, and which worked in practice.

Occupational genesis as a model for the delivery of health care might very well have been addressed earlier, if occupational therapists had been able to articulate its underlying premises with confidence. This may be the ideal time to articulate such a theme, for the economics of health care raises questions as to whether the structures of modern health delivery are able to meet society's needs (Starr, 1982). Might an awareness of occupational genesis contribute to the sound economics of graded, adaptive living, meeting society's health care needs along with the needs of the individual? To develop this concept further and demonstrate its worth through research would meet the goals of the pragmatists and social activists who conceptualized and formed a profession to enable individuals to move towards health and function, so that they might be contributing members of society.

Summary

Although the pragmatists, Dewey, Mead, James (Serrett, 1985c) and Peirce, provided a foundational philosophy for the profession, the relevance of pragmatism was not made known to the profession, apparently due to interpretations made by its founders in regard to the education of therapists; no study of philosophy was incorporated in the education of occupational therapists. This lack of foundational material later led to attempts by numerous occupational therapists to devise variously labeled philosophies, theories and models of occupation. Yet these attempts did not wholly encompass all aspects of practice, nor resolve questions the profession has had about itself.

Occupational therapy's explicit adoption of the foundational concept of occupational genesis would permit the themes of neurodevelopment, systems theory, group theory and activities to be synthesized under the philosophy detailed by the pragmatists. With a holistic philosophy devoted to the healthful development of the individual and society through automatic and purposeful, active occupation, the profession could devote itself to demonstrating its value in meeting society's needs, by meeting the unique needs of individuals.

The Magic of Healing

Occupational therapy was built on an important basic premise: activity promotes healing. This notion dates back to biblical times and has been repeated throughout history in many sources. Yet, this is a difficult phenomenon to explain, and a creative skill to deliver. Activity serves as the basis for a profession devoted to healing mind and body.

A colleague and I describe occupational therapy as magic. That is the only logical rationale we can give for a set of activities that have such profound effect without apparent explanation. We describe the use of scooter boards in improving reading skills, and scratch our heads in explaining their relationship. While the relationship between sawing and filing wood and increasing strength is clearer, it does not explain why one is willing to endure pain and resistance for longer periods than in doing straight exercise. There are many other unanswered questions associated with activity.

Our students are very willing to believe in our explanation of occupational therapy as magic. Their own experiences with activities strengthen those beliefs. Our classes are supplemented by an activity laboratory that includes activities that range from clay to computers. It does not take much time before our students report a visceral reaction to our laboratory. For some, it produces intense anxiety and frustration; for others, it is a respite from the drain of other academic pursuits that clearly makes them feel better. And the physical well-being that accompanies enjoyable activity is well documented.

Even with these experiences, it still is sometimes hard to believe that activity is a tool for healing, especially when one works within the medical community. After all, where is the science in occupation? Why does one activity have a positive result for one patient and no such reaction for another?

We live in a world that reinforces these questions. The public seeking pills, CT scans, surgery and other serious medical interventions may well ask, why is that therapist offering me yarn, or paint or other such stuff? What will making a basket do for one's health?

The answer is, perhaps nothing. Perhaps making a basket is not the healing tool for you. But something is. And that's the job of the occupational therapist – to find the right tool.

Maybe a time will come when we will be able to be prescriptive in our approach to therapeutic activity. But I suspect not. Learning to approach healing with the right tool requires a professional approach, not a technical one.

Following are some articles about healing that span a variety of topics. I am sure they will remind you of the magic that you experience every day in your own practice.

Engaging the mind to help the body overcome illness

Originally published in *Advance for Occupational Therapy* Jan. 23, 1995

Occupational therapy students know that the minds and bodies of their patients work together in the rehabilitation process, but they sometimes ask me how they can attend to both in an activity-based treatment program. I tell them the story of Elizabeth.

The 76-year-old woman lived alone in a suburban New Jersey community her whole adult life. She suffered with severe rheumatoid arthritis for many years and reached the point where she was totally unable to care for her own needs. With no family to help her and her funds depleted, she was admitted to a nursing home which was to be her permanent residence.

I found Elizabeth severely debilitated. Her constant pain and the disease process had left her with severely restricted movement in every joint in her body. Believing she could not perform even the slightest activity on her own behalf, she was totally dependent, and her depression was pervasive – all the more so because she had retained every bit of her intellect.

Elizabeth was clever, interesting and witty, with a biting humor. In addition she was meticulous, albeit she had little control over the latter except as she could meet this personal need for order through the actions of others, which sometimes caused friction between her and the staff. I saw her fussiness as a strength upon which she could call, and approached her with interest and respect.

We began a two-pronged approach to therapy. Elizabeth's first goal was to feed herself. Mine was to engage her in an activity program that would increase her upper-extremity range of motion and pain tolerance to permit her to achieve the goal. Toward these ends, I constructed a splint for her right hand, which was so deformed that she was unable to use her fingers in any functional way. The splint was designed to stabilize her fingers and wrist, and at the same time, hold a spoon or other utensil.

I had a number of discussions with Elizabeth about the kinds of activities she might be interested in, and the ways we would approach these things to help her become more mobile. We decided on weaving because it was the only thing she could physically do.

I knew it would require a great deal of effort on her part because of the pain she would undoubtedly experience. But Elizabeth had a goal which I knew the craft could facilitate. 'This will help you feed yourself,' I told her. Expecting only that from the effort, she agreed to participate.

A small frame loom was warped and set up with clamps in front of and toward Elizabeth's right side so she could reach it. The weft yarn was pre-cut so each row used a separate length of yarn, leaving fringe at each side. I taught Elizabeth how the yarn went over and under each warp thread, but she was unable to grasp the yarn and pull it through.

As it happened, we were in the process of fitting the splint during this time, so we adapted the splint so it had a small projection on the medial aspect adjacent to the MCPs. This projection took the shape of a miniature crochet hook. Now we had a tool Elizabeth could use to weave with as well as to eat.

And weave she did. At first, slowly and painfully, but then picking up speed, Elizabeth became a masterful weaver. Her meticulous nature came to the fore. Her weaving was precise and beautiful. She had an eye for color and began to weave creative patterns. Her work was such than many of the staff would bring her yarn, and she would work up pillow covers for them for a small fee.

Needless to say, Elizabeth was very pleased with her success and the attention she was getting for her work. Moreover, the movement that came with her activity was precisely the movement she needed to feed herself. She became independent in feeding. With this gain in independence, she was less of a burden on the staff, who responded by treating her more sensitively. And she in turn became more patient with them.

I wish I could say that Elizabeth made even more progress, but the extent of her disability was such that she was limited in achieving further gains. I can say with certainty that the activities of feeding herself and weaving made a significant change in her life. They gave her dignity and a sense of pride in her accomplishments, and they contributed positively to her relationship with others.

Without the motivation, skill and increased tolerance for pain her weaving provided, I doubt that Elizabeth would have gained the range of motion she needed to become independent in feeding.

Students are amazed to see the arts at work in the clinic

Originally published in *Advance for Occupational Therapy* March 20, 1995

Each year students and former students come by or take the time to write to tell me about some craft they used in fieldwork or in their new practice and how therapeutic it was. They all seem very surprised to find that an art they learned in class is actually used in the clinic. Although I usually tell the students that our class offers a selection of activities commonly used in the clinic, and that we chose these arts because they are so often seen there, they just don't seem to believe me. Many are amazed when they first see these activities being used as therapy. Invariably my response to them is, 'Why am I not surprised?' And we laugh.

Every once in a while one of the students tells me a story that really illustrates the value of these arts in therapy. Karen Roston was so impressed with her experience that she wrote me when it happened, and we talked more about it when she returned to school the following year.

Karen had volunteered as an occupational therapy aide during the summer between her first and second years of occupational therapy school. She had completed her activities courses, but had not worked in a clinic before. On her first day at the hospital, as she was standing and sorting some materials, she overheard the therapists describing a new patient who would be coming into the clinic. This middle-aged woman had had a mastectomy and was now experiencing severe edema in the arm ipsilateral to the mastectomy. In addition, she was depressed and debilitated. The therapists were trying to envision which activity might be appropriately therapeutic. Something that required her to keep her arms elevated would be ideal.

Karen thought, 'Macramé would probably work,' but she kept the thought to herself as she was not yet fully familiar with medical conditions, and she was uncertain as to how an occupational therapist should approach this problem. To her surprise, she heard the therapists say, 'Macramé probably would be a good activity. Too bad our last student left. She knew how to do it.'

Then one of the therapists turned to Karen and said, 'You're from the same school as our last student. Do you know how to do macramé?' When Karen said yes, the therapists asked if she could teach the patient.

Karen investigated the closets. She found some suitable cord and a D-ring used for splinting, and she was ready. But when the patient came into the clinic, she was far more debilitated than Karen had imagined. The young aide had no idea the woman would be in a wheelchair. Her posture was poor; she was obviously depressed and in pain. She was unkempt and barely communicated with the staff.

The project Karen had planned, a plant hanger, clearly was not suitable for this patient. It required too much strength and range of motion. Karen quickly rethought her plan and adapted to the circumstance. She set the woman up with a bracelet, a project with shorter strings that required less strength. She placed the project so the patient would keep her arms elevated as she worked. The patient quickly learned the technique and soon could work unsupervised. And as she worked, Karen noticed that the edema was diminishing, just as they had hoped.

When it was time to leave, the patient wanted to continue working at home. Karen made up a kit of everything she would need, put the items into a plastic bag and sent her on her way. To Karen's surprise, when the patient returned she had completed her projects, her edema was gone, and her attitude had changed. She was bright, alert and enthusiastic. She began to make bracelet after bracelet, including beads in the design, and was soon selling them to hospital workers and friends.

The change that macramé had made in the patient astonished Karen. The woman now stood erect and walked tall. Her mindset was positive, her appearance neat; and she was productive and proud of herself.

Karen is a convert to crafts as therapy. I understand from her friends that she is taking as well as giving courses in crafts in the evenings. And I'm quite sure she's using her ideas in the clinic as well.

Why am I not surprised?

In times of bereavement

Originally published in *Advance for Occupational Therapy* March 13, 2000

On Jan. 19, a tragic fire broke out in a freshman dormitory at Seton Hall University in South Orange, NJ, where I am program director. Three young men were killed in the fire, and many others were injured and displaced. One of the pre-occupational therapy students escaped injury by running out of the smoke-filled building. A third-year master's degree student was on affiliation at St Barnabus Hospital, spending some of her time in the burn unit where many of the injured were taken.

After the initial shock, and despite fear about the welfare of friends and classmates, our occupational therapy students said, 'We want to do something to help the community heal.' One notion was to set up an area on campus where students and faculty could create get-well and sympathy cards. Students had learned through lab activities that creative arts elicited feelings and offered meaningful opportunities to express those feelings. The students wanted to share this understanding with their friends on campus.

It became evident to the faculty that these students had learned the value of active occupation as a healing force.

People engage in many different kinds of activities when they are confronted with bereavement. Each faith and culture has its own rituals. Many cultures have rituals that seem foreign to others but are meaningful to those who participate. Some mourn briefly before burial and extensively afterwards, governed by prescribed rituals and timeframes. For others it is the reverse. A somewhat lengthy period in which the deceased is 'waked' marks the mourning period, and with the burial, the formal mourning period ends.

During the mourning period, prescribed rituals often dictate the clothes people wear and how those clothes are treated. In some cultures, black-colored clothing signifies mourning, whereas for others the wearing of white prevails. For some the rending of clothing symbolizes loss. Gender roles often dictate behavior; some cultures have extreme taboos in this regard. In some cultures, flowers mark grief, while in others, starkness is in order.

Meaningful prayer takes many forms and is expressed in all cultures. Some prayers are said individually, some are mandated within a group. Traditional prayers have traditional implements. (Prayer beads such as the rosary are used as part of such ritual.) The sense of community that prayer builds around people who are mourning is important to their recovery.

Food plays an important role in bereavement rituals. Whether it is the casserole brought by caring neighbors or the boiled egg that represents the unending cycle of life and death, eating has a healing quality. It is something to do together, and it assures that the deep depression mourners feel will be countered by something pleasant and by the care of friends and family who use this opportunity to see to their loved ones' welfare.

In some cultures, children are excluded from bereavement rituals; in others, they participate. When my own mother died, I was deeply comforted by the fact that each of my children and grandchildren, down to the littlest ones who could perform this task, placed a shovelful of earth upon her coffin. This ancient tradition in which we all participated brought the family together and brought us together with our ancestors.

Meaningful activities that are shared have deep healing qualities. Going through old photographs can be helpful as can sharing humorous memories of times with the deceased loved one. For some, it's important to sing. Writing eulogies or memorial poems is another way to mourn.

At Seton Hall, our classes are very diverse, giving us the opportunity to explore cultural differences in mourning practices. One of the activities that we will do in our adult development class this spring will include a sharing of these notions of grief. I usually have the students work together in small groups and share their families' death rituals. It may be particularly meaningful for us to deal with these issues this term, given the tragic losses we have experienced.

Each year, as we discuss these death rituals, we bring to students' attention the fact that they will be losing patients, often unexpectedly. The attendant loss is painful and must be dealt with. We advise the students to find groups in which to talk about their losses. Sometimes they can do that in the workplace, but sometimes it is not available there. Religious leaders and others can help.

We encourage students to call each other, and to call upon faculty, because sharing grief is an important part of the healing process.

Don't overlook some handcrafts for your rheumatoid patients

Originally published in *Advance for Occupational Therapy* Sep. 16, 1996

Today, people are coming to increasingly value handcrafts once again, as they recognize the mind–body connection and its implications for health. There has been a corresponding resurgence of the use of traditional occupational therapy media in many clinics. However, some therapists are unprepared to introduce such media, due to their own lack of experience. Their hesitancy is understandable, since some activities that may appear therapeutic in fact are not.

One example of a potentially detrimental activity for a patient with rheumatoid disorders is knitting, even though it may seem useful on first analysis. Knitting requires that the needles and yarn be held in a static hand grip, which is more apt to produce stiffness; as the project grows, it can provide a steadily increasing weight which is apt to cause strain on the joints of the shoulders and arms.

But there are media more suitable for treating the rheumatoid upper extremity. Doing crafts also can teach these patients skills that have application to their life roles. They are aided in succeeding when they learn to develop adaptive approaches to activity planning and performance.

Clay, although it's a resistive medium that may be contraindicated for damaged joints, can be made less resistive by adding water. Pinch pots encourage finger flexion and opposition. On the other hand, coil pots encourage finger extension along with shoulder flexion/extension and elbow flexion/extension. This kind of exercise may be more useful for certain patients, especially when used in combination with tools with built-up handles.

Sanding greenware in preparation for glazing is very appealing to many patients. Beads of clay are fun to make, and sorting and stringing them requires fine motor skills.

Reeds need to be soaked in water to make them flexible enough to be made into baskets. While reed is ordinarily worked out of water, the weaving can be done in a warm-water bath, combining treatments. All the fingers are involved in dextrous and individualized movements during the weaving process. Working the reed is fairly non-resistive, but this, of course, depends on the weight of the materials selected.

Weaving yarn can offer different degrees of shoulder range of motion, depending on the size of the loom. The larger the loom, the more movement is required. A small frame can be warped for exercising the fingers. This activity can be adapted many ways to meet individual needs. For example, using short strands is less demanding than using long ones. Macramé is made by making knots of various descriptions and arranging them in different patterns. It is easily adapted to be large or small, long or short, to make either plant hangers or friendship bracelets, for example. Macramé can be hung from above, encouraging shoulder flexion, reach and shoulder abduction, along with grasp. The resistance can be managed by using different materials: jute requires more strength to tighten; light yarns are easily made taut.

There are many types of paper crafts. Paper-folding (origami) offers one of the few really good finger-extension activities; painting can be widely adapted in position and medium, using hands, brushes or palette knives. Collage is good for encouraging group interaction and personal expression.

Woodworking is a resistive activity good for building strength and range of motion. Sanding blocks can be adapted to restrict hand movements into desired positions, such as by using a dowel in a block to place the hand into a neutral pronation/supination posture.

Food has universal appeal. Its more generally valuable activities may include tearing lettuce for salads, kneading bread, or rolling pie crust to provide exercise. Learning new food management techniques may be important for someone who needs to reduce energy output while maintaining responsibility for the family's meals.

Games, of course, should be part of the therapeutic repertoire if for no other reason than that they are fun. There is some evidence that the immune system is affected by emotions, so managing and expressing emotion may play a role in handling autoimmune diseases such as rheumatoid illnesses.

How activity affects your patient's recovery process

Originally published in *Advance for Occupational Therapy* June 17, 1996

Recognizing where one can help patients adjust their activity profiles requires an openness to patients' likes, dislikes, values and culture. It is all too easy to make recommendations for an activity that seems logical from one's own personal perspective, but may indeed be contrary to a patient's needs, capabilities and preference. Activities are not easily prescribed. Just as someone may agree to a prescribed medication in the doctor's office and not comply once he is back home, so it is with activities.

When therapists' suggestions and patients' lifestyles are in conflict, it may be difficult to resolve the cognitive dissonance. To be a better therapist, recognize the meaning of an activity in the individual's life, and your own role in aiding that person toward healthy activity.

Activity requires movement, thus pain management is a constant consideration for patients and therapists. On the other hand, activity can mask pain. Each involves both mind and body. Activity requires the integration of the two in performance, and understanding that integration can be a tool for pain management.

The integration of mind and body elicits two interacting phenomena. One, the body moves as the mind concentrates on that movement. Or, as the mind is engaged, the body can perform automatically.

We all experience these phenomena; they are particularly evident as we learn new skills. For example, when learning to type, we must search out the letters and struggle to make fingers reach the near and far keys. But once the skill develops, our hands move freely from key to key while our minds create thoughts. Once the movements are fully automatic, we perform them with total unawareness of finger placement. We sometimes even remain engaged in tasks beyond the point at which we might ordinarily tire, if the work is compelling.

The same sequence applies in learning to ride a bicycle. Once we do not have to concentrate on coordinating leg and trunk movement, our attention is diverted to the destination. Mind and body interact to make these choices, and to perform with skill, ease and effectiveness. Satisfaction occurs when performance meets our expectations.

Concentration of the mind during movement of the body plays a significant role in pain management and reduction, particularly for those with rheumatic diseases. And pain reduction facilitates secondary joint mobilization. Anecdotal evidence abounds of individuals who report their willingness to tolerate activity well beyond what they could tolerate in rote exercise.

Were it not for the interest otherwise afforded by slot machines, for instance, one would be unlikely to sustain this repetitive movement for the hours players spend at the task. One occupational therapy department in Nevada installed a slot machine in the clinic. Needless to say, it was a busy piece of equipment.

The cultural relevance of activities lies in how they fit with the commonly accepted activities of the society in which an individual lives. In the United States, we live in a culturally divergent society. There is room for many kinds of activities, some of which are relevant regionally or in terms of gender, age, family customs, or even current style. What is meaningful to one group or at one point in time may be less meaningful for others at other times.

Selecting activities requires skill in activity analysis, skill in the analysis of functional performance, and a full understanding of the disease process. Activity analysis rests on a comprehensive understanding of the many features each activity provides and their potential effects on patients. Such analysis provides one with the ability to recognize similarities and differences among activities as well as their patient for eliciting change. The activity's motor requirements, the cognitive ability needed to perform the task, and the inherent affective qualities all enter the picture.

It is also necessary to know the tangible components of any activity, as well as its interactive effects, because human beings do not act in isolation. They need tools, environments and others with or for whom to act. A comprehensive activity analysis is composed of hundreds of items.

Analysis of functional performance requires a full understanding of the individual's physical and mental capabilities, and his or her potential within the constraints of the disease process.

Activities must be meaningful to patients or they will not engage in them. Individuals differ widely in their interests, so one must be careful in selecting or recommending a therapeutic activity. It cannot be approached as other scientifically based treatments because they elicit individualized responses.

Yet one underlying generalization can be made. Mobilization through activity is best achieved when the individual engaged in the task finds it sufficiently interesting.

A patient loves to do the teaching

Originally published in *Advance for Occupational Therapy* July 15, 1996

We tend to approach therapy with the assumption that the therapist is there to help the patient to learn. And most often, that is the case. However, sometimes the best therapy comes when the patient is able to help the therapist learn – that is, when the patient sets out to teach the therapist a particular skill.

One patient of mine was a genuine expert in food preservation, even though dementia ruled most of her existence. One day while we were working together in the kitchen preparing a salad, I casually mentioned that my garden was overflowing with tomatoes, and that I really didn't want to have to can all that produce. I often babble to patients about things related to home, because I think patients need to hear about real things.

This woman, who had always seemed confused, told me that I could freeze the individual tomatoes and that I didn't need to do any canning. When I asked her to explain, she told me I should just place the tomatoes on a cookie tray in the freezer, and when they are frozen slip them into a plastic bag and store them there. Then when

I wanted the tomatoes for cooking, I could take them out individually and run them under warm water to slip their skins.

I was somewhat skeptical, because I was uncertain of this woman's cognitive abilities, but because I had so many tomatoes, I thought I could risk one. So I cautiously put one tomato into the freezer overnight, and removed it in the morning, expecting who knows what to have happened. Well, lo and behold, it worked; the tomato was as pretty as a picture, and I could use it for anything I wanted to cook.

Now I perceived this woman in a totally different way. She knew it, and I knew she knew it. Her ability to solve my problem made her understand that I valued her knowledge and experience. She grew more through teaching me than she had from my teaching her. And I surely grew as well.

I have found that the best way to build self esteem in patients is to allow them to show me how to do things. I have learned woodworking techniques from a vocational education teacher who was an acute psychiatric patient. I learned sewing, magic tricks and card games from hand and spinal cord injured patients. And I learned incredibly creative ways to get off and on the toilet from patients with hip fractures, strokes and amputations.

Not only can patients teach therapists, they can teach one another. My colleague Liz Lannigan recently told me a story about two young patients with whom she worked several years ago at a psychiatric clinic in New England.

One young man, let's call him John, was in his mid-twenties; the other, whom we'll call Bill, was in his mid-teens. Relying on her experience, and a sense that they would be good for one another, she set the two of them to a task together. John was experienced at woodcrafts, and Liz asked him to show Bill how to put a kit together. The two young men both seemed to enjoy the experience.

Several years went by and Liz was working at another hospital in the area. One day the receptionist call to say she had a visitor. She was surprised to find John standing there. She asked him why he had come. He reported how meaningful he had found his experience at the hospital, where he learned the rewards of teaching someone else. And he wanted her to know that he had turned that positive experience into a career. John had become an occupational therapy aide in a home for youngsters with special needs. He attributes the fact that he found a meaningful life vocation to his occupational therapy experience.

Surely these are still the things we seek today, despite the restrictions imposed by new service delivery options. We should be looking for such opportunities, and I believe if we do, we will find them.

A hard look at reality

Originally published in *Advance for Occupational Therapy* Aug. 12, 2002

I had the wonderful opportunity to visit Stockholm, Sweden, and the World Federation of Occupational Therapy Congress earlier this summer. At the conference, I met Ann A. Wilcock, the author of *Occupation for Health*, vols. 1 and 2. Volume 1 deals with the history of the use of occupation as a tool for health. I was very impressed with the extensive research Dr Wilcock did, and was left with a very positive impression about our origins, and the intelligence of medical personnel in their approach to healthful living and recovery.

When I returned home, I visited one of my colleagues who had had knee replacement surgery and was experiencing rehabilitation, including occupational therapy. But the practice my friend was exposed to bore no resemblance to the practice Dr Wilcock describes. Actually, it bore no resemblance to anything that I recognized as occupational therapy.

Not once was my friend asked about her life needs. No therapist inquired about and knew, for example, that her office was on the upper floor of her home. She is a single parent, and no one inquired about any parenting experiences she might have difficulty with. The only reference to home was the acknowledgement that there would be no homecare, based on the diagnosis she carried. That she could plan ahead for limitations she would experience was apparently not considered, with one exception.

A small group of post-surgical patients were assembled to talk about the kitchen. However, no active occupation in this environment took place. And because my friend was an experienced therapist, she noted several ideas that were not even suggested. No mention of rolling carts; no demonstration of reachers. Just talk. Patients' questions remained unanswered. The therapists were assigned large notebooks in which they were to fill out forms in a constant mode of reporting, and no activity to report about.

More frightening than what I observed about my friend was the observation made by another patient, who asked my friend, 'What do occupational therapists do?' In order not to bias her, my friend responded, 'Tell me what you think an occupational therapist does.' To her horror, she heard, 'I think they are equipment sales people!'

Interestingly, my friend swears that the occupational therapist assigned to her did not know her name, even upon discharge.

Unfortunately, my friend later had a serious fall, sustaining an injury that has caused her pain and restricted her recovery. One has to wonder. Did the quality of her 'rehabilitation' contribute to her fall? It seems to me that these occupational therapists are either poorly trained or have succumbed to the rules set out for practice by some superior with a vision or motive that is inconsistent with the principles of occupational therapy. Occupational therapy cannot be provided unless there is active occupation. Has therapy become so rote that professionals are not needed? The impression that patients are getting about their rehabilitation may be closer to the truth.

If you are working in a facility that advances this quality of practice, you should think long and hard about your own participation. There are other options. If you cooperate in reducing occupational therapy's quality of care, then you are part of the problem. Just because an insurance company is paying for the service doesn't make it occupational therapy!

Letter to the Editor:

Is reality in the mind of the beholder?

Originally published in *Advance for Occupational Therapy* Sep. 9, 2002

After reading 'A Hard Look at Reality' (Activity Notebook, Aug. 12) one wonders: 1) how long it has been since Estelle Breines has seen the inside of a rehab clinic and 2) how the occupational therapists she reports on (or, should one say, 'butchers') would have described the same events.

Ms. Breines' column is long on criticism and short on suggestions for improvement. How, for example, can the therapist have assessed 'parenting experiences [the patient] might have difficulty with,' set appropriate goals for this, and documented the treatment in a manner satisfactory to reviewers for Medicare or other third-party payers?

How can the therapist have performed an evaluation that accounts for all such minutiae and completed all the necessary documentation for such an evaluation and still conformed to the productivity levels her facility or company requires?

The very suggestion that the quality of the therapy this patient received may have been responsible for her subsequent fall is not only scathing but unsubstantiated.

So who really needs to take a hard look at reality?

(Correspondent, OTR/L)

Editor's note: Since the patient herself was an OT in this instance, it is unlikely that she misinterpreted and therefore misstated the treating therapist's actions to Dr Breines. See Activity Notebook for a full answer to this writer's two important questions this week on page 7. [See article on next page, 'Don't "learn" occupational therapy from unfriendly sources'].

Don't 'learn' occupational therapy from unfriendly systems

Originally published in *Advance for Occupational Therapy* Sep. 9, 2002

It isn't often that I have the opportunity to respond to a reader's comments about what I have written, but I appreciate the opportunity whenever it presents itself.

I wrote Aug. 12 about the rehabilitation experience of an occupational therapist who moved over the line from therapist to patient. In that column I reported what I had been told, not only by the therapist/patient but by other therapists who visited and spoke with her as well. I commented on the shocking lack of active occupation the occupational therapist/patient received – to the point that her roommate thought occupational therapists were medical equipment salespeople!

A patient is a whole individual, not a diagnosis. A patient is composed of mind and body, lives in a tangible world of time and space, and relates to others in significant ways. Together, these influences interact and are brought into play in the active occupations in which all humans engage. This is fundamental Occupational Therapy 101.

In a letter this week, Maryland therapist M.F. questions, 'How, for example, can the therapist have assessed parenting experiences [the patient] might have difficulty with, set appropriate goals for this, and documented the treatment in a manner satisfactory to reviewers for Medicare or other third-party payers?'

The only way I know to begin to find out is to ask patients what their lives are like, what problems they anticipate, and go from there. Unfortunately, some of the finest, most reputable institutions have so systematized the rehabilitation process that the individual uniqueness of the patient is removed from the process. I think their intentions are good, but they have taken the wrong tack. Good therapy will pay for itself. Short-sighted economy will not.

Bright young therapists seek jobs in prestigious facilities to gain experience, and learn to work in these restrictive environments under the impression that this is state-of-the-art practice. My contention is that good therapy can and is being delivered in places that allow more attention to be paid to unique patient needs. I know this from personal as well as secondary experience.

The current focus of insurance payers is function and functional improvement, and they have tied this to reimbursement. That is the reason that physical therapists are trying so desperately in legislative efforts throughout the United States to incorporate function into their scope of practice. Occupational therapists have always had a clear understanding of how to assess function, and creatively return patients to former (or at least improved) levels of function. We must not lose this skill. The caveat 'use it or lose it' takes on additional meaning here that has implications for our profession. We must recognize the economy associated with functional performance. The fully functioning person costs less to support, and in fact contributes to the support of society.

Is the question how to document change? That's the easy part. Virtually all function is measurable in some form or other. You can count minutes of endurance, numbers of items moved, etc., speed or performance, etc. What should be counted? It all comes down to what has come to be called the 'narrative'. The Canadian Occupational Performance Measure (COPM) is a tool that relies heavily on the narrative. If we were treating a body part alone, we would not need the narrative. But we do not practice that way. An occupational therapist must take into consideration the personal lives of patients, assess how a disability interferes with performance, provide an occupational approach to the restoration of function, measure change and report it accurately and with lucidity, so the reader (insurance company) understands what the process has been and how the therapy contributed to the gains.

If you are being asked to deliver practice that you do not value, try to change the procedures so they better meet patients' needs. If you've tried and were unsuccessful – if you are being required to work in a way that does not meet your patients' needs – find another job. I have walked away on two occasions from positions that I felt were untenable. One of my former students has just done the same.

While I recognize that there are some areas of the country where the job market is not terrific, there are lots of areas where the jobs are plentiful. Remember, occupational therapy is portable, both geographically and in the sense that we can easily move from one area of practice to another. It may mean that you will have to learn some new skills. But none of the skills you already have will be wasted.

Treat yourself the way you would like to be able to treat your patients – with dignity and support – and move on.

Letter to the Editor:

Originally published in *Advance for Occupational Therapy* Oct. 7, 2002

I am a rehabilitation manager in a large acute-care hospital, and articles such as [Estelle Breines'] allow me to convince our team of OTs that occupation-based practice is not only possible but essential for the survival and prosperity of our profession.

At times those of us who espouse this view of practice are seen as dinosaurs or 'Ivory Tower' thinkers. I can tell you first hand that we have had success at our hospital in implementing a conceptual model of practice (the Lifestyle Performance Model) completely re-doing our evaluation and treatment processes as well as our competencies and activity inventories.

This occupation-based focus is difficult at first but leads to much greater patient as well as staff satisfaction. I believe that acute-care OT is one of the most difficult areas [in which] to implement such practice, but once successful, [it] can have the most impact.

... Thank you, Dr Breines, for continuing your work and your writing of Activity Notebook. You have my support in any way, both in fieldwork settings and possibly in any research editorial submissions! I frequently require my staff to read your articles ...

Michael Amory, MS, OTR/L
Program Manager Dept of Physical Medicine & Rehabilitation
St Luke's Hospital
Bethlehem, Pennsylvania

Old Crafts, New Ideas

When I was first enrolled as an occupational therapy student, it was clear to me that I would be taking lots of classes in which I would learn how to do a variety of crafts. I not only learned ceramics, woodworking, metal crafts, paper crafts, yarn and fabric crafts, printing, jewelry making, plastic crafts and something called minor crafts, but I learned to analyze and apply them from every perspective.

Most of my classmates were very good at these manual arts. In fact, a propensity for handwork seemed to be what drove our interest in the profession. For me, it was my love for crafts along with my love for science and health that brought me to occupational therapy.

In time, the curricula became filled with more and more theoretical material and many schools began to eliminate crafts from the occupational therapy program. At first, there was an expectation that students had many of these skills before they enrolled and so it was not necessary to teach it in school. Craft knowledge was treated as a prerequisite. Later, as the clinics themselves began to eliminate activities in favor of exercise, the rationale to reduce the craft content of occupational therapy education was reinforced. The result has been the graduation of occupational therapists well trained in theories and in science but with few skills in the performance of activities.

Some networks of interest in the use of active occupation remained and struggled to retain the crafts in educational programs and in clinical settings, but it has been an uphill struggle.

At one point, I was asked to write some articles to illustrate to young and inexperienced therapists how activities can be applied as clinical tools. I have come to recognize how important these examples are. Just today, I read a message on a list serve from a young therapist asking for suggestions for providing hand exercise in the home. While I was initially astounded that one could be a graduate occupational therapist and be so limited in one's knowledge, I was immediately reassured by the many answers that came winging back across the ether. Apparently, there are still some therapists out there who are competent, knowledgeable, creative and effective.

The articles included in this chapter describe a variety of crafts that can be used in multiple ways to meet therapeutic needs. They include paper crafts, bobbin lace, painting, knitting and other activities. There is also an article that makes the case that most crafts stemmed from the trades and are examples of how tools of work that developed in former times have evolved into leisure tasks in the modern era.

In sum, it must be noted that many of the public are actively engaged in these sorts of activities, creating a thriving industry and that, although they do not meet the standards of scientific rigor, they are certainly meaningful to the people who ultimately become our patients.

If you haven't got any steel, try using some papier maché

Originally published in *Advance for Occupational Therapy* Aug. 21, 1995

At the WFOT Congress in London last year, I made a startling discovery. A gentleman from Zimbabwe demonstrated adapted chairs, tables, wheelchairs, standing tables and the like, made out of papier maché.

I examined samples of his items and could see how incredibly sturdy they were, even though they were made out of paper. The Zimbabwean assured me that these items were not apt to mildew or deteriorate, even though they were put together with flour or rice paste and other such materials.

Such homemade technology has made it possible for his patients to have equipment they could not have had under any circumstance. In addition, the clients who participated in their construction had painted them with colorful designs. Some were quite beautiful.

One of the most useful and least valued items in the clinic is probably paper. We take it for granted because it is so abundant, and we are so accustomed to seeing it as part of the trash stream. Not everyone feels as we do. When I visited Israel several years ago, I saw how zealously paper was conserved there. Israelis use tiny scraps of it for note taking – and they use both sides.

Papier maché can be a very useful tool for the clinic. I recall a group of parents who constructed a large piñata for a children's holiday party. They built the papier maché around a box, building it up to the shape they wanted. The project took several sessions to complete, as it had several steps and needed to dry. Before the piñata was completed, the group poked a hole in one end and filled it with candy and small toys they had made, then they sealed up the hole with the strips, let it dry, and painted it with designs.

At the party each of the children had a turn swinging a bat at the piñata until it broke, spilling all the goodies about. I can't tell you how satisfying this experience was for the parents and children alike.

Papier maché can be made in a number of ways. Although the pulp is commercially available, the easiest and cheapest way to make it is with strips of newspaper torn to about 1 inch width and 10 to 12 inches in length. Dip the strips into a solution of paste that can be made from flour and water or any white glue and water. Place the strips onto an armature or base of some sort. The base serves as a structure for the project and therefore determines the shape of the finished project.

You can build the strips up to whatever thickness is desired, allowing the work to dry between layers. After the project is finished and dry, you can decorate it with paint and glaze it with shellac or polyurethane.

Papier maché is a very popular material for making puppet heads or dolls. You can construct the head on any round form. Once it is dry, cut the papier maché in half, remove the form and reseal the halves with moistened strips. Or you can use a balloon as the base form. When the paper is dry, the balloon can be pricked with a pin and the shape will hold.

Leave a small hole at the base. Paint the head in any style. Attach a cloth bag – shaped to represent the arms and body of a doll – to the head with a ribbon and glue, leaving the bottom open to accommodate a hand. The hand is inserted into the bag with two fingers placed in the arms and one finger in the hole in the base of the head to control the puppet's movements.

Not only is puppet-making fun, but puppets are very useful tools for expressive play, both for physically and mentally impaired patients. People are often able to express feelings through puppets that they are unable to express directly.

Another fun project is to make imitation vegetables and fruits from papier maché. Fashionable but costly if you are to buy them in the stores, these decorations are very inexpensive if you make them from scrap paper. Eggplants, cucumbers, pears, apples are easily made; artichokes are a little more difficult. Construct the form of plasticene, and reseal the halves. The only trick to making the fruit realistic is to carefully match the colors. Activity analysis of this project reveals that it uses several hand skills: pinch, reach, gross and fine-motor performance and cooperation also come into play.

By working together, each one doing aspects of the tasks he or she can effectively perform, the group can produce a number of different fruits and share them among the workers. Or the group can offer them as gifts or sell them to generate income for a favorite charity.

Chasing Belgian lace

Originally published in *Advance for Occupational Therapy* Aug. 20, 2001

Several years ago when the World Federation of Occupational Therapy conference was in London, I extended my visit to see some more of England. During that trip through the English countryside, I ventured into Bath, a beautiful and interesting city that dates back to Roman antiquity and beyond. In my travels, I went into a local yarn shop. I seem to go into yarn stores in every city I visit, since yarn crafts are my favorite leisure activity. In fact, I usually return home with yarn or needlework, or at least a book with directions and patterns. In Auckland, New Zealand, real wool country, I bought beautiful books on knitting. In Lake Tahoe, I bought yarn and instructions for making a felt hat.

While roaming through the store in Bath, I came upon bobbins for making bobbin lace. I couldn't resist and bought an instruction book and a bunch of bobbins. When I returned home, I learned that I would also need a special pillow, which I wasn't able to find anywhere. The age of the Internet had not yet arrived. I also discovered that this was one craft that I couldn't quite figure out from the book alone. So the bobbins lay in a bedside table for these many years.

This summer I was planning a trip to France, and it occurred to me that now was the time for me to find out how to do bobbin lace, as the French are renowned for their lace making. I was determined to go to buy my special pillow. However, a friend of mine with whom I was traveling did some research and suggested I would do better to go to Belgium and take a class there. Belgian lace is also famous, so this seemed like a good plan. France and Belgium are neighboring countries, and traveling to them both would make my trip more interesting. My friend found a school in Bruges and we worked our schedule around the French and Belgian national holidays so we could see both the lace making school and the celebrations.

Bruges is one of the most beautiful cities I have ever seen, with remarkable architecture and winding canals. It was built around 1100 AD and everyone must have decided it was a place to keep secret to preserve it. Neither my friends nor I had ever heard anything about it. Finding a class in this medieval fairyland was a real treat.

The participants in the lace making class were all women I estimate to average about 70 years of age. One woman who was able to converse in English had been coming to this class for 29 years, and advised me that bobbin lace is her hobby. It would have had to be a hobby. She was finishing up a lace tablecloth that had taken her five years to complete, and she showed me pictures of the one she had completed five years before. No wonder the prices of Belgian lace were prohibitively expensive.

I watched very carefully, and finally understood how this remarkable craft is done. Each project has anywhere from 20 to 100 bobbins hanging from it. The bobbins are tossed over one another in an intricate pattern that reminded me of miniature macramé. Keeping track of the pattern requires tremendous precision. Some of the women were beginners and needed help from the teacher, but all of them were experts by comparison with me.

One thing that I noticed was that the special pillow they use in Bruges is different from the style used in Bath, and is particularly large, flat and round, about 24 inches in diameter, with a wooden backing. The Bath style pillow is cylindrical, about 10 inches long and about 5 inches in diameter, firmly packed with batting. This pillow is used to support the work, and to place straight pins into to keep the pattern as one works.

When I went to the school's shop to discuss my purchases (another book, more bobbins, special pins, Egyptian cotton), I expressed my reservations about dragging such a large size pillow on a trip that required us to carry everything we owned on and off trains. The shopkeeper said, 'You don't need to buy the pillow. Just use Styrofoam™ until you decide you like to do bobbin lace.' If I had only known that before!

So here I am, back at home, with nothing to stop me. My plan is to begin the simplest project and see how it goes.

I guess the moral of the story is the importance of leisure activities that continues to be meaningful throughout one's life. Here's an activity that is so interesting, so compelling, so beautiful, that generations of people continue to pursue it, developing increasing skill as time goes on. These women come together to work and learn, much the way women have always gathered to do crafts together. Quilting bees are a prime example of this sort of group activity that holds tremendous meaning for the participants. Even though time passes and technologies change, there seems to be a continuing need for people to join together in creative activities. There is something very meaningful in joint and purposeful efforts, especially when there is a product to be created. And there is a continuing need throughout life to gain new skills or refine others. Remembering the importance of learning and creating throughout life is a belief that occupational therapists hold with. Seeing the values of these ideas being sustained by dedicated women is a genuine delight that I will never forget.

Letters to the Editor:

Originally published in *Advance for Occupational Therapy* Oct. 15, 2001

I enjoyed your article ... and thought I might share my bobbin lace experiences ('Chasing Belgian Lace', Estelle Breines, Sept. 17). I'm a British-born OT, currently working in Memphis, and I, too, love 'yarn crafts' as you call them. I lived in Spain for

22 years – in fact I did my occupational therapy training in Madrid. While living in San Sebastian, I went to a class run by a local school of art on bobbin lace ('encaje de bolillos' in Spanish). This was something I had always wanted to do. I bought the equipment, learning from my teacher that each country uses slightly different types of pillows and bobbins. I agree with you that it is quite difficult! I made a strip of lace, about one inch wide, using (I think) 64 bobbins, and it took me about three months to make a strip about 18 inches long. I always intended to make it longer, and use it to trim a baby's sheet or something, but I think it got lost when I moved to the United States. In any case, I have forgotten how to do it!

Because of my interest in the Spanish language, I went on vacation to Puerto Rico in 1999, and decided to drive to a town called San Sebastian (same as where I used to live). There, I found that the art of lace making was thriving! There are several old ladies still making lace, and I bought several lengths of lace trim and one handkerchief, all very reasonably priced. I sewed one piece onto the bottom of a plain white curtain, and it looks very pretty.

By the way, the art of lace making is almost lost in Spain; the teacher I had was about 65 years old (this was 15 years ago), and she had learned how to do it at age 7 from a very old lady. She was very good. Just thought I'd share these experiences with you. Most people here have never heard of bobbin lace!

Juliet Phillips, OTR
Memphis, Tennessee

When I read Dr Breines' article it immediately brought to mind a picture I saved from a magazine many years ago which was a copy of the painting 'The Old Lacemaker', by Nicholaes Maes, showing an old woman asleep next to her bobbin lace. The caption underneath says, 'In therapy as in art, mastery is distinguished by the response produced.'

I thought this was a timeless description of occupational therapy.

Ruth Levy, OT/L
Staten Island, New York

If Martha has them doing crafts...

Originally published in *Advance for Occupational Therapy* Dec. 15, 1997

As many of you know, Martha Stewart has a television program and a magazine in which she teaches viewers how to do various crafts, cooking and gardening. Stewart reports that she received 2.2 million hits on her website in its first month – and according to *USA Today*, she has 3 million viewers on her new daily syndicated shows. That's an incredible record for any public figure. But it seems all the more remarkable for someone who advocates crafts.

I wondered with some mirth: what if we changed the name of our profession to the Martha Stewart Therapists? Would that make us more prominent? More acceptable? More valuable?

I have been a dedicated Sunday morning watcher since I first discovered her show. Not long after I did, I began to hear pseudo-sophisticated comic references putting down her approach to activities. After all, the crafts she demonstrated were so 'foolish'. Some of these comments were made on the media, some I heard at dinner table asides. Martha Stewart had become the symbol for silly women who like to waste their time doing crafts. It became pretty slick conversation to make a snide remark denigrating the skills Martha demonstrated.

But one day I noticed that two young women I know – one an MD, one a college educated business manager – were subscribing to Martha's magazine. Still no talk of the virtues of 'doing' seems to be confronting nay sayers. Apparently, people are reading and watching in private! Millions of followers value Martha's premise that active occupation is meaningful and satisfying.

It still seems odd to me that so many people are supporting this woman's ideas in the privacy of their homes, while public comments about her remain negative. She is criticized both for her aggressiveness in business and for the topics she shares with her public. Is this dual criticism a form of anti-feminism? No matter. She survives and thrives.

What is there about our society that prevents people from coming 'out of the closet' as craft fanciers? Clearly we are in conflict about our values. Martha has proven that there are many passive recipients of these ideas. But few individuals have spoken out about the value of the projects she undertakes.

So here we are – a profession grounded in similar beliefs – yet failing to take advantage of our skills in these media and failing to glorify our abilities to use these media to establish health in our clients. It seems to me there is an enormous need in our society for people who can demonstrate skill in crafts, so that they can become meaningful aspects of the lives we live.

Perhaps the popularity of Martha Stewart's programming is a sign that the pendulum has begun to swing back from a perspective that promoted science and devalued arts, to one in which society is demonstrating its interest in the value of meaningful activity. Martha Stewart and Bob Vila are cashing in on this knowledge. Isn't it time we did, too?

Every time we succumb to the pressures – sometimes more imagined than factual – of insurance managers and HMOs, we are heading in the wrong direction. Active occupation leads to health. We are well qualified to demonstrate that premise. Our job is to make it possible for our patients to lead meaningful lives by enabling them to participate in the kinds of occupations that bring them health.

If Martha and Bob's people are finding it meaningful to engage in active occupations that extend the purpose of their lives, we should remember that these are the very same people whom we ultimately treat.

By eliminating the use of active occupations from our therapeutic repertoire, we eliminate the tasks that people find meaningful, and therefore deny ourselves and our patients the right to fill their time with things that lead to healthful living.

If our society is turning toward acceptance of meaningful activity, and demonstrating that by supporting such activities, we should heed the message. If activity is healthful in wellness, it can certainly be healthful in illness. This is a direct message from the founders of our profession.

If we have to think of ourselves as 'Martha Stewart therapists', so be it. But I think it's enough just to think of ourselves as occupational therapists.

Paint can be all-purpose medium in the OT clinic

Originally published in *Advance for Occupational Therapy* June 16, 1997

Paint is a great medium for therapy. It can be used in so many ways, and has so many interesting qualities.

We usually think of painting as an expressive activity which allows for symbolic representation. It can do this for both the individual and the group, and the medium lends itself to both parallel and collaborative tasks.

During fieldwork, one of our students set up a painting activity with a group of detox patients. Each was given a set of written directions designed to help with sequencing problems. The student hung a picture for the group to copy.

They set to work with great interest. Quite naturally, each painting looked very different, even though they were copying from the same picture. Following the activity, the works became the focus of a discussion group. Working together on the same project seemed to be a catalyst for merging group members and helping them communicate, both with one another and about their own special problems.

Paints themselves have varied qualities. Oils, acrylics and water colors act differently on paper and actually can be used in different ways on different kinds of surfaces. Oil paints require more time, but oils, because of their opacity, can be painted over to alter the picture or achieve different visual effects. Oil paints lend themselves to long-term projects because they take a long time to dry.

On the other hand, water paints need to be worked quickly. They commit themselves to paper and cannot be reworked easily, because when one tries to rework them, one gets a muddy result, and even the paper can become damaged.

Depending on your goals, it is important to select your media carefully. For selected paints, be sure to use the correct brushes. It's amazing how many varieties of brushes there are. I strongly recommend a visit to an art store to see what sorts of items are commercially available.

Paints have broader applications than as paper and table tasks. I have always found working on a group mural to be an excellent therapeutic tool. People's behavior patterns are quite evident when they work together on a project.

In addition, because of the symbolism that emerges through creating something, mural painting tends to reveal to both therapist and patient a great deal about underlying issues of concern. Certainly it provides an excellent opportunity to provoke discussion. And if you can paint on a real wall, all the better.

In fact, my favorite painting experience had nothing to do with art or creative expression, but it had a great deal to do with meaning. I was working as the activity consultant to a small private nursing home in northern New Jersey, where the patients had most of the traditional activities one sees in nursing homes. But there was a small cadre of elderly men whose interests were not being served by the program being offered. The men were belligerent, uncooperative and ornery – to everyone. Needless to say, most of the staff didn't want to go out of their way for this bunch. But I felt that their active belligerence said they still cared; they wanted some control over their lives and some meaning in those lives.

So I put them to work. I hauled in paint cans, rollers and brushes, and with a little urging, they were off to a room that needed a new look. The patients who could stand painted high; the patients in wheelchairs painted low. And the maintenance man did the ceilings and touch-ups. For once, a little pride had entered their lives.

I've also had patients paint old furniture and do stenciling – a very easy thing to do and very effective. While you can easily make a stencil from old X-ray film, there are lots of commercially available stencils in the hobby shops and catalogs. Hold the stencil firmly against the object you are decorating, and use a stiff brush or a sponge to dab paint on the cut-out areas. Carefully lift the stencil and move it along to the next spot to be painted. Repeat the process until you are finished.

Use the appropriate paint for the project you are doing: latex wall paint for walls, oil-based paints for furniture. With this medium, you are limited only by your imagination.

With knitting, you can be teacher or student

Originally published in *Advance for Occupational Therapy* May 18, 1998

I received a gift for the holidays from my grandchildren – a book that had instructions on how to knit the cutest hats! The most wonderful idea was in the book. It appears that most sweaters take the same number of stitches that you need to make a hat, so you can take unfinished sweater backs or fronts and convert them into hats by stitching the seams together and decorating them with ropes and pompoms and such.

As I have been knitting since I was a child, I have an unending supply of left-over yarn. Perfect for making hats. And the children love getting them as gifts. I ran to the drawer, pulled out two half-started sweaters, and quickly turned them into hats. One went to my daughter, who likes to ice skate, and one I gave to my students to raffle off for the student fund.

I was having such fun finishing these projects that it reminded me of an Australian wool sweater project I never finished. I had bought the yarn when I was in Australia for the WFOT conference eight years ago. The yarn was three different colors, having been sheared from sheep which were naturally white, black and gray. That was what had compelled me to buy it. I had started to make a cardigan with irregular color swatches, but never finished it. Maybe this time I will.

Knitting is a very comforting occupation. Depending on your level of skill, there is something for everyone. It is an activity that most people who have the use of both hands and reasonable cognitive ability are able to learn. At first it takes a great deal of attention, and the beginner is apt to drop stitches or even add some. It takes a bit of investment in learning to knit accurately and automatically.

Knitting consists of two stitches: knit and purl. Each is the reverse of the other. By combining these stitches in various ways and learning to shape the work, you can complete a number of projects.

And there is something very satisfying about making oneself a knitted garment or making a gift for someone else.

I remember when my 11-year-old son decided to make my daughter a scarf for her 13th birthday. I will never forget the surprise and delight she expressed when she received it, and the pride Ric felt in having completed such a welcome gift.

There are lots of memorable sweaters, socks, mittens and hats I can recall. It seems as if I knitted memories along with the yarn. Shades of Mme. Defarge. There was an English teacher in college who made me stop knitting (in class) the gift I had planned for my fiancé. I was so worried about getting it done by his birthday.

There were funny mittens I made, with space for my index fingers. And the baby buntings that each of the children got to take their babies home from the hospital.

Some of the students asked me how we use this craft therapeutically. After all, knitting is a skill that takes time to learn and the current health care environment is not filled with time. It seems to me the best way to use knitting in therapy today is by letting patients who can do it teach you how.

Many times, what a patient needs most is to feel valuable. The people with whom we work are so often suffering from feelings of despair, accommodating to their disabilities. What is of critical importance is to generate feelings of worth in damaged souls.

And you can take pride in having encouraged the patient to take pride in self.

Buying craft supplies tells something about the users

Originally published in *Advance for Occupational Therapy* April 15, 1996

I am always on the lookout for new craft ideas and new sources of supplies. I do this partly to keep up with what's new out there so I can include these items in my class, and partly just because I love 'stuff'.

I love to wander the streets of Manhattan on my way to work, taking a different route each day. The best part of my day is spent peering into the windows of all the little shops as I wind my way downtown through the fabric district with all its yard goods, ribbons and laces, into the bead center with its strands of unusual beads from all around the world, through the jewelry market with findings and clasps for junk and precious jewelry, and best of all, through the dollar stores whose merchandise can never be predicted.

I live in a rural community in western New Jersey, where these items are not available in the same way. Still, there are other pleasures in the country.

Yesterday, I took one of my periodic pilgrimages to a major suburban craft supply center. One of the things I noticed is that people of all ages were shopping for crafts. Also, I realized that very few of the materials on sale were much different from the craft supplies that I used when I was in OT school.

This didn't surprise me, because there are only so many materials that can be worked by hand. For example, there's clay, wood, metal, plastics, leather, fabrics and yarn, all of which are found in stores today. But there are almost unlimited ways in which these materials can be used and some of the new applications are creative and very simple.

I noticed that lots of the techniques that I know how to do with simple materials were boxed up expensively. For example, a simple weaving loom that can be made from an old frame and woven with inexpensive bulk yarn is presented in packaging with quantities of poor-quality material that inflates its costs prohibitively.

Moreover, all too often the items, once produced, result in a tacky product. For the same effort and less cost, these same techniques could be used to produce very beautiful, well crafted items.

I also noticed in the store that many of the items were pre-cut for easy assembly, and the selection was enormous.

This is a far cry from the time when every item needed to be individually cut. We've come to realize in this time of managed care that having therapists spend time for preparations is prohibitive, so finding attractive pre-cut materials is welcome indeed.

Yes, there were lots of kits in the store, but there were an equal number of bulk items from which one could select. I was very pleased to see this, because choice is such a critical feature of creativity, and for some patients, choice-making is a skill that needs to be learned. The bins of colored beads, paints and other baubles were wonderful to look at, and fun to touch. My family had to urge me that it was time to leave. I didn't leave kicking and screaming, but I felt like it.

So, why do I bring this to your attention?

I think that occupational therapists can learn from this. If people are buying these items, in kit or bulk, of wood or leather, costly or cheap, young and old, they must be getting something out of it. 'Plain, ordinary' people find crafts interesting and meaningful! Certainly, this must be true, or these huge craft centers would not be able to sustain themselves. These centers are not diminishing, they are proliferating.

Not too long ago, if I wanted to find cord for macramé, for example, I had to go to my local hardware store and it came in one color, ecru. Now there are colors and materials galore, along with glues and stuffing and all other manner of craft items.

If the public is using crafts to an ever-increasing extent, shouldn't we look at what it is that interests them about crafts?

We live in a society that is increasingly slick, with plastic money and automated work and play, more often watched than engaged in. This kind of world reduces the amount of creative energy and personal control that used to be a part of everyday life. I think that people are returning to crafts because it allows them to reintroduce these elements into their lives.

Many of our patients are missing these very same elements in their lives. Whether they suffer from physical or mental deficiencies, they may need a little help in learning how to resolve these issues. The occupational therapy practitioner can help patients lead satisfying lives by using crafts in therapeutic ways. One way to start is to go shopping. I'll bet you won't want to leave the store either.

Quick! Find the knitting needles!

Originally published in *Advance for Occupational Therapy* Oct. 29, 2001

It's been a long time since I knitted anything, but knitting was my first craft. I learned how to knit from my mother, who always had needles in her hands until the end of her life. She could read and knit any pattern and others came to her to learn, myself among them. I became a master knitter, but lost interest after time. The children had grown, my drawers were full of sweaters, my office was too warm, and fashions had changed.

Some of my earliest memories revolve around knitting. As a child during World War II, I can remember how my mother knitted sweaters for the sailors. There was some distribution center in the community that provided the yarn. I was so young at the time that I never figured out where the yarn came from, but come it did. There was a never-ending supply of yarn, and we produced sweater after sweater.

Women in the neighborhood chose either khaki or midnight blue yarn to work on, and this was their contribution to the war effort. My mom always chose midnight blue, because she had a brother in the navy who served on an oil tanker in the Pacific, and the knitting made her feel close to him. And as this was my favorite uncle with whom I lived, it made me feel close too.

Because navy was hard to see, fewer people chose to knit that color yarn, preferring the khaki. This was never a problem for Mom, as she could knit without looking. Needless to say, I learned to imitate her and soon learned to knit without looking as well.

It was our family's habit to go to the movies every Friday evening. Well, Mom and I took our knitting with us. Mom would knit the complicated parts, like casting on, doing the ribbing, forming the shoulders and sleeves. She gave me the body of the sweater to knit, which I could do more easily. So we sat together in the theater, knitting away and feeling productive, knowing that our work would be keeping some sailor warm. We got tremendous satisfaction from our work, not to mention the attention we got from our neighbors in the theater.

On September 11, 2001 we entered a war, not of our choosing, but a war nonetheless. My immediate recollection was the similarities to my experiences during WW II, which I shared with my students, because I did not know what else to tell them. What rational person could understand what had happened to us?

I'm sure I don't have to describe how this disaster made me feel. Everyone was feeling the same way. Lost, angry, uncertain, frightened. For some reason, I found myself drawn to a yarn shop while visiting my older daughter's home in Cleveland. There, I immediately decided to make a prayer shawl for my youngest daughter who is a cantorial soloist in the Boston suburbs. It was important for me to create something to give away, particularly something of a symbolic nature. This was not something I had planned, but I was compelled to select yarn, invent a pattern and begin. When I picked up the needles, the strangest calm overcame me. I knitted constantly until I finished the garment, realizing as I worked that the knitting was helping me to heal.

Some of the crafts that were traditional have remarkable qualities that we have tended to overlook in recent years. Even in our media labs, we have eliminated knitting, and have very brief approaches to other crafts, being sensitive to the current health care climate. Our students ask us about the practicality of what we are doing, even as they learn to love many of the activities. But in reducing our attention to traditional activities, I think we have lost something that could be very helpful.

We are now in a time of extraordinary stress as we continue to hear about events over which we have no control. Bombings, anthrax, fear about opening the mail, fear of flying, traffic restrictions in and out of New York City and Washington, long lines at airports with repeated identity checks, etc. I wonder if we should examine the usefulness of some of the traditional crafts that have offered meaning and satisfaction in the past to see if these can be of help now.

Recently, I have heard of some interesting events. People are telling me that renewed interests in knitting have started up. Public figures are seen knitting, and lunchtime knitting groups are being formed, joined by men as well as women. Some years ago, Rosie Greer's fondness for needlepoint started a nationwide hobby. Perhaps there are other crafts that could be identified as helpful to the public's mental health. I think I'll put up a sign offering to start a knitting group, as my contribution to the war effort. Some things never change.

Crafts were the basis of the trades we still practice

Originally published in *Advance for Occupational Therapy* Dec. 16, 1996

If we examine active occupations from an anthropological, historical perspective, we may come to a deeper understanding of crafts.

Before the advent of tool making, hunter-gatherers used their hands to survive. Whether they lived in the tropics, on the savannah, in the desert or in ice-covered lands, human beings had to learn to manipulate the flora and fauna around them to produce the resources they needed to sustain them. Basket-making, clay sculpting and making objects out of leather were among the earliest human skills.

As people used these skills, they became more inventive and more adaptive, devising hand tools to further their abilities. Flint knives, pounding tools, and lances were refined into myriad other tools.

Creating and using these new things furthered human understanding of how the elements in the environment could be altered. So people were then able to create new materials such as metals, which in turn created better tools. Skills in tool use expanded exponentially throughout the world. Weaving, woodworking and metalworking developed.

Invention expands into industry, and soon into new technological skills. Ancient humans adapted their skills to their lifestyles, and their lifestyles in turn modified the skills. As they evolved, all the activities in which groups of humans engaged melded into cultures, with the newest activities replacing the old in terms of societal value.

Today, as in the past, the old activities remain, but the new ones seem more important because they mark change and enable new development.

All crafts require skill. They are actually the basis of all the trades. Masonry, carpentry, jewelry-making and other occupations are skilled crafts still used by society to meet its needs for survival and artistic expression.

For crafts to have meaning, they must contribute to someone's welfare; they must meet people's needs. Crafts are valued when they allow people to contribute to meaningful events in their own or others' lives.

Artistic expression is one type of meaningful event that imbues satisfaction to people. It enables the individual to communicate with others in deeper ways.

Another meaningful event in people's lives is satisfying personal desires. When one needs an object that will enable him to function at a higher or more meaningful level, and he can create that object, the satisfaction established is expressed as competence or efficacy.

Still another meaningful event in human lives is satisfying the needs or desires of others. Creating something that others find meaningful satisfies a personal need. All of these purposes are important in occupational therapy practice. Each can be employed in conjunction with the use of crafts.

Whenever people use crafts to meet personal needs or desires, to meet the needs or desires of others, or to express themselves in expanded communication, they will find the crafts as meaningful as human beings have always found them.

If, however, the activities chosen offer no personal meaning, they belie our heritage as human beings and occupational therapists.

Use crafts, but use them with discretion. Do not use them if their purpose is not clear to you, when they waste either time or effort, or when their product does not instill pride and satisfaction.

Crafts are the occupations that got human beings to their current level, and there will be new crafts to emerge that will bring us into the future.

An attempt to define purposeful activity

Originally published in *American Journal of Occupational Therapy* 38: 543–4.

An initial look at the term *purposeful activity* suggests it would be difficult to define except in terms of the individual. Because purposeful activities are unique constructions for individuals, the term eludes definition as a conceptual whole.

Elude, however, does not mean defy. To elude is to hide, to evade exposure. That the profession of occupational therapy has only recently attempted to synthesize a consistent and official definition for purposeful activity (Hinojosa, Sabari, Rosenfeld, 1983) despite a history of repeated use of the term, is evidence of this elusiveness.

In the past, the use of purposeful activity in treatment has been debated. This discussion often centered on the meaning of the term, with therapists taking opposing positions as to those modalities and activities that they considered appropriate to practice. I, too, shall enter the debate and attempt to examine the term *purposeful activity* by addressing issues that underlie the problem of achieving its definition.

A first step in definition is to analyze each word in the term. The dictionary defines purpose as 'an end to be obtained, intention, determination' (*New Britannica/Webster Dictionary and Reference Guide*, 1981, p. 736.). Activity is defined as 'vigorous or energetic action, liveliness, a process that an organism participates in or carries on by virtue of being alive, a similar process actually or potentially involving mental function' (p. 10). These definitions, when seen in light of one another, reveal that personal will is integral to the understanding of each word. Further, individual intention and choice are inherently related concepts, both to each other and to the concepts of personal will. Finally, purposeful activity suggests both mental and physical involvement. Thus, the mind/body unity to which occupational therapy subscribes correlates with the term that has long been associated with its practice.

Philosophical origins

The educational philosopher, John Dewey, expressed the concept of purposeful activity before the occupational therapy literature. In 1916, Dewey proposed that occupation is conceptually allied with purposive action inherent in play and work (Dewey, 1916). He believed that development was structured by independently constructed striving, relevant to the individual's personal explorations. Dewey also proposed that the elements of personal choice and self-direction are enabled by active occupation. This concept is among Dewey's principles that appear to have been adopted and adapted by occupational therapy's founders toward application in health care, which is not inconceivable considering their historical relatedness (Cromwell, 1977; Dykhuizen, 1973). Although the occupational therapy literature does not refer to pragmatism, it does demonstrate it. Therefore, Dewey may represent the basic philosophy upon which occupational therapy is based.

Discussion

Arguments within the profession about defining the role and tools of occupational therapy have centered around the use of purposeful activities by occupational therapists. Because there had been no official definition of the term, the need for definition increased as the profession moved from its conceptual origins toward wider health applications. As these practice vistas have expanded, it has become less clear to therapists how to deliver practice and retain their unity and identity as occupational therapists.

Several authors represent various positions around which the argument has been drawn. Fidler (1981) addresses the value of tangible creations and interaction toward increasing the patient's self-image. Similarly, Huss (1981) asserts that action upon environment defines occupational therapy. Yet her view includes associated neurodevelopmental principles and techniques, a dimension absent from Fidler's view of practice. Huss goes on to address the use of mechanistic modalities and rejects their use for occupational therapy. In response, English et al. (1982) refute this position, defending the use of such modalities in practice. Certainly it is common knowledge that therapists in all dimensions of practice differ widely in their use of tools. Those just mentioned represent some of the variety of views occupational therapists have expressed in practice.

In analyzing these positions, it seems evident that occupational therapists define their practice by the tools they use (Mosey, 1981) rather than by the process in which patients engage. Therefore, the arguments about definition may reflect therapist role identity conflicts rather than conceptual foundation criteria. A profession that adopts a concept of mind/body synthesis must reach beyond the tools of the therapist to reflect on the motivation or intent of patients as they engage in living.

Occupational therapy is not what therapists do to their patients. It is a collaborative effect of therapist and patient directed toward eliciting cognitive/perceptual capacities of patients through development of skill in all levels of performance (Breines, 1981). Therefore, purpose or purposeful action cannot be defined in terms of the tools with which, or activities in which, therapists engage their patients. Purposeful activity must be defined in terms of the unique directions of individual patients and the enabling of patients toward enhanced growth and development, and by involvement and organization of self and environment, both structural and personal.

Using these parameters for definition, all activities requiring both mental and physical involvement in which occupational therapists and their patients engage collaboratively can be assumed to be purposeful activities, if they elicit choice and provoke development. It is the occupational therapist's role to identify and ameliorate or circumvent barriers to that development. The goals must be those of the patient. Goal-directed activities assume intention and purpose on the part of the individual. It is also the therapist's role to identify will and barriers to will, assuming that with all life there is will, although perhaps not the will idealized by the therapist.

Choice, intention, or purpose are not always in conscious awareness (Hofstadter, 1979). The occupational therapist can serve two roles regarding choice or purpose. One role is to bring patients' intentions beyond choice and into automaticity. Automaticity is defined as behavior that occurs without conscious awareness. For example, proprioceptive neuromuscular facilitation and neurodevelopmental training can be interpreted as a means of solving praxis disorders through clarification of antigravity discontinuity. Praxis or motor *planning* reveals an element of choice or intention in its expression. Conscious attention, or planning, is an indication that skills are being attempted, but automaticity in performance is a sign that skills have been achieved. To be able to perform skillfully requires the ability to disregard, and disregard is enabled by automaticity. Sensory integration is directed at increasing spontaneous responses as a means of eliminating barriers created by the necessity to choose among behaviors. Moving behavior from conscious to below conscious awareness and into automaticity is viewed as enabling.

On the other hand, in the second role, the therapist may be directed toward bring patients' automaticity to conscious awareness. Group tasks that highlight interactional patterns and the use of media to elicit symbolic representations are such examples.

Issues of personal intention, occupation, and relationships associated with development were of concern to early twentieth century philosophers outside occupational therapy (Dewey, 1916; Mead, 1932). Occupational therapy appears to have adopted these principles and applied them to health care.

Much attention in the education and practice of occupational therapists has been directed toward the technology of practice and away from these early principles. This attention to tools has clouded our understanding of the pragmatic principles of personal choice upon which our profession was founded. The dispute in our profession about tools is founded on an illusion, perhaps facilitated by the medical model by which we have been directed, which is leading us away from the educational and philosophical principles upon which I suggest we were founded.

Conclusion

I conclude that purposeful activity cannot be defined by one individual for any other individual, other than that it requires both mental and physical involvement. It is a personal construction, which is solely dependent on individual choice and subject to the influence of the structural and personal environment of the individual; this position is consistent with the philosophical principles upon which the profession probably was founded. Further, it may not be valuable to stress the tools of occupational therapists; rather, the developmental process in which our patients are engaged should be emphasized. With this emphasis, the tools must follow, as I believe has been demonstrated by our current admirable level of practice, which is founded on a sound philosophical heritage.

Acknowledgment

Ann C. Mosey, PhD, OTR, FAOTA, is acknowledged for having stimulated the discussion cited here in her course in Advanced Occupational Therapy Theory at New York University.

Toys and Games

My favorite lecture of the year focuses on defining the terms toys and games. Each year, I divide the class into two groups. I ask one set of students to make a list of every toy they can think of, and then to organize the list in a developmental sequence starting from earliest childhood and going on. The other set of students is asked to do the same task for games. They start off slowly, but pretty soon they each have a lengthy list. While the answers vary from year to year, for the most part the toys range from mobiles through bicycles. The games tend to begin with peek-a-boo or clap-hands and go on to organized sports.

This opens the opportunity for me to describe toys and games in terms of occupational genesis. Toys are features of the environment (the exocentric realm). Games have rules, and usually require more than one person, so they fit into the consensual realm. Now some games, like solitaire, have rules and only require one person, but the fact that there are rules seems to qualify them as consensual, since people play the games according to set rules. As a matter of fact, in our family solitaire is a group game because everyone feels free to 'kibbitz'. For some games, there are 'table rules'. That is, the group playing the game agrees to the rules, and the rules can change to meet the needs and wishes of the group.

According to these categories, toys are tools to be manipulated. In fact, they are often elements of games. Games, on the other hand, demonstrate social communication skills. Of course, toys and games can just be fun, but that is not usually why occupational therapists are concerned with them. We use them to increase sensory, motor, cognitive and social skills.

The articles that follow are limited to just a few kinds of toys and games, but the idea of using toys and games as therapy is much broader. A good background of acquired skills in play activities, both for children and adults, expands the repertoire of the therapist. It is a great excuse for sitting down to learn a new game or to build your skills at play. Remember that when you need a break!

That perfect task may be in the cards

Originally published in *Advance for Occupational Therapy* Jan. 22, 1996

The other day I asked my friend Beth Torcivia what her favorite therapy activities are. She shot back, 'I can do anything with a deck of cards, two balloons and a rubber band.'

After we both finished laughing, I thought of my own days of running between home health clients, nursing homes and school systems, often all in the same day. The back of my car looked like the remnants of a garage sale. I never knew who the next patient would be, and the nearest clinic was usually miles away. I had to rely on the simplest of materials, and use them in the most creative ways.

Just like Beth, one of my favorite tools was a deck of cards. It fitted in my pocket and could be called on for all kinds of purposes. To this day it is still my favorite evaluation tool, for it can reveal so much about a patient's assets and deficits.

I will never forget the seriously emotionally disturbed middle school student referred to me, who could not focus on academics. He and I played War until he learned which numbers were higher and which lower. Using a game not only made learning possible, it improved his ability to manipulate objects.

A deck of cards can be sorted by color, suit and/or number. Sorting can be graded in complexity, and switching from one mode to another is a perceptual/cognitive task that can be enhanced with practice. Having an individual lay out a Solitaire sequence can tell you a great deal about his or her recognition and memory, either recent or past. Playing Go Fish is also good for identifying memory and recognition skills (not to mention Bridge, for the more sophisticated among us).

Solitaire is appealing to many kinds of people. Knowing a number of different versions of Solitaire games makes it possible to draw upon them selectively for remediating various problems. Many of my hand and stroke patients with hand involvement enjoyed playing Solitaire. It was something they could practice when they were alone.

Solitaire can be a competitive game as well. Double Solitaire requires two players, and cognitive speed as well as dexterity helps one to win. There are often two patients with similar or different disorders who can benefit from playing double Solitaire together. It can also be a good activity for family members seeking something to do with patients.

Laying out the cards and playing the game is also a good activity for someone with a mild visual field cut. Patients can be instructed to use compensatory head movements to aid them in developing new skills in tracking.

Learning-disabled children with spatial orientation problems often enjoy playing with cards. While on a rocker board, the child can pick a card from the deck and put the spades to the right, the hearts to the left, the clubs in front and the diamonds behind. Working on balance and placement together can be fun.

A variation on the proverbial 52 Pickup is to place cards in an array around a young patient who is either seated at a table or on a mat. Just reaching to pick up target cards can increase range of motion, balance, dexterity and grasp-release.

Mix two different decks together and have the patient sort one from another. You can vary the complexity of this task by using different colored decks or same-colored decks with different designs. Or mix two identical decks together and have the patient create two full decks from them. This, of course, requires planning, counting and sorting skills.

How about making a house of cards? Is your own patience up to it?

Just shuffling a deck of cards is a great dexterity exercise, particularly if you bend the cards into one another to create a 'bridge'.

Now, about balloons and rubber bands...

Cards are well-suited to therapy goals

Originally published in *Advance for Occupational Therapy* Jan. 8, 2001

When one is raised as an only child, as I was, learning to play alone becomes an important skill to develop. Our family had a copy of Penguin Hoyle which had the directions for every card game known. On rainy days, I would take the book out and teach myself any number of games. My favorites, of course, were the various solitaire games. I learned a number them and would turn to them when I was alone to fill the hours.

One game of solitaire in particular struck my fancy, and became a source of great interest long into my adult years. This game is played with two decks of cards and is very complex. In due time, everyone in my family became expert in this game. My mother played it every evening in her widowhood, and it was a great companion to her. My children all learned the game as well.

As members of my family learned the game, an interesting thing happened. It no longer was a game played alone. Because of the complexity of the game there are many choices of moves, and everyone adopted their own style of play. As soon as someone set out the cards, everyone else gathered around and had something to say about the play. It seemed that one could view the options better from the side, so having a companion comment on the game was often helpful. Disputes did come about, but the companionship of the decision making was welcomed by everyone, and everyone recognized that the player had the last word.

One year during the holidays, I received a wonderful gift from my son. It was a computer disk with a game on it. Magically, the solitaire game that had amused my family over the years was now a game for the computer called Arachnid. This game, whose origins had been lost in time, now had a name. It has a home on my laptop computer and comes with me on trips to while away the hours of travel. It is never boring, and is a well loved friend.

Card games are variable in complexity and format. Analyzing these games for their various qualities can turn them into great therapeutic tools. For example, a wide array of cards may be a problem for a patient with a visual field cut. That wide array may help the patient remember to turn his or her head to compensate. Some games require counting, enhancing cognitive memory. Alternating colors and building from low to high call on still different perceptual skills. Other games call for planning ahead.

So pick up a book of card games and learn some yourself. They will expand your therapeutic repertoire as well as provide a new set of leisure activities for yourself. And if you want to know how to play Arachnid, read on. Just remember, it takes many hours of play to learn this game, and you will win only rarely. But when you do, you will be delighted, and you will probably be hooked forever.

Mix two standard decks together. Deal 10 cards, face down and separate from one another. Repeat three more times on top of the first ten cards, totaling 40 cards in 10 stacks. Deal one card each onto the first 4 stacks. Deal the next 10 cards right side up on each of the stacks. There are now 54 cards dealt. The object of the game is to place cards in a sequence from ace to king in each suit. You may move any card onto any other card regardless of color or suit. You may move any number of cards of the same suit together onto any other card. You may not move cards together that are of different suits. If you move a card and reveal a down-facing card turn the down card face up. You may move any card into an open space. If you move a king into an open space, you cannot move it out as there is no place to put it. It is best to try to gain as many open spaces as possible, as this will permit you to move cards in and out of the space to manipulate the play. When you cannot make any other moves, deal out an additional 10 cards on top of the others. That will make the array very complex and will require a great deal of planning and problem solving. Good luck!

Here's an easier one that uses one deck. Count out 13 cards, placing them face down. Deal 1 single card above and to the right of the 13. Deal 4 cards, one under the single card and to the right of the 13, and three more to the right. The single card is the base number card. For example, if you have dealt a 3, all 3's are to be placed alongside the first 3 and will serve as the base for each suit. A 4 is placed on the 3, a 5 is placed on the 4, and so on. An ace is placed on the king, a 2 on the ace. When 3 through 2 are played in one suit, remove the suit. The cards are manipulated so that reds and blacks are alternated. When you are unable to play any cards, turn over three cards from the pile left in your hand, repeating until the deck is finished. Then repeat. This is a little tricky, but fun. Enjoy!

It's all in the cards

Originally published in *Advance for Occupational Therapy* April 2, 2001

I received a wonderful note from one of our readers. Sharon Newton, an occupational therapist, is a captain in the US Army. She wrote the following memo to me, and I thought it would be fun to share what she had to say:

'I am writing about your recent column ['Cards are well suited to therapy goals', Jan. 8]. I, too, have often used a deck of playing cards as a therapeutic modality. Besides the obvious use for fine-motor skills, I love what cards can do for cognitive skills as well! In fact, I am currently with a combat stress control unit ... Needless to say, I don't carry a lot of fancy assessment tools with me when I go "to the field", which is where I really get to practice my craft. A deck of cards fits nicely in my cargo pocket, and it provides a wonderful screening tool for me to assess a soldier's cognitive function.

'I have them play a game of Concentration, which allows me to observe immediate recall, following directions, etc. The interview [is] less threatening, because we aren't just sitting across from each other with me asking them questions. Anyway, I just wanted to share my experiences, and to say that I look forward to your articles. Keep it up.'

Needless to say, I was delighted with the positive input, but more than that, I am thrilled to find that occupational therapists who have available to them the most up-to-date equipment are using simple tools to ascertain functional capacity. This is not only economical and informative, it is good occupational therapy.

It was also very interesting to me to learn about a modern military application of occupational therapy. I think that those of us in the civilian world tend to forget the important role of occupational therapy in the military. Occupational therapists have worked with military personnel since the outset of the profession. Our literature talks about the origins of occupational therapy in the mental health arena, but too often forgets the role of the military in its earliest development.

Military personnel were treated for both physical and mental disabilities. I have a vivid recollection of photos of bicycle saws that were used for strengthening the lower extremities while patients engaged in purposeful activities with the arms and minds.

Some of the most creative occupational therapy was provided to patients by therapists who served these populations. In the earliest years, these occupational therapists functioned outside direct military appointment, but served in the United States and abroad in military hospitals treating their patients. After a time, the occupational therapists received military commissions, and served the patients and their country with honor.

It is encouraging to read that this tradition still continues. These well-trained therapists provide service to their patients with a clear understanding about how to use activity meaningfully. It makes me feel proud to be associated with them. Thank you, Captain Newton, OTR/L, for bringing this to my attention.

How about getting all 'dolled' up?

Originally published in *Advance for Occupational Therapy* Nov. 17, 1997

I had the pleasure of visiting a private pediatric clinic the other day, where I saw some wonderful papier maché doll heads that had been made by children Claire Daffner was treating.

Besides these colorful projects – made from paper bags, paint and sparkles – there were some magnificently crafted soft sculpture dolls that Claire herself had made. Some of these were several feet tall, carefully stuffed, dressed in beautiful clothes and with remarkable character revealed in their faces.

Clearly, here is a therapist who understands the value of dolls in eliciting self-expression. Moreover, her own creativity revealed that dolls can be meaningful for people of many ages. Remember, our homes are decorated with images of all sorts, made of all sorts of materials.

Claire's dolls reminded me of the fun I used to have making marionettes from simple dolls, using tongue depressors – a craft I learned in occupational therapy school. Or the dolls I used to make as a child, from old socks – a craft I later taught my children and still later, my grandchildren. This surely is a timeless activity.

I wonder if we have forgotten some of the old techniques that children once found meaningful, having replaced them with technologically advanced items made of hard plastic or electronic gadgetry. Revisiting some of the old toys children used to enjoy might be very therapeutic. Children do not discriminate in their pleasures. They like the old as well as the new.

Not only do children enjoy making dolls, but making dolls for children is something adults enjoy as well. Depending upon the goals for treatment, the dolls can be made of soft materials such as fabric and stuffing or from wood, which needs sawing, sanding and painting.

Here are some simple 'recipes' for dollmaking:

Papier Maché Puppet/Doll

medium-sized brown paper bag
newspaper
flour
water
toilet paper roll
tempera paint
glitter
felt-tip markers

Tear the newspaper into one-inch strips. Mix the flour and water to a consistency of glue. Stuff the paper bag with crumbled newspaper (this will be the doll's head). Secure the paper bag to the toilet paper roll with glue. This can be a handle or it can be secured to clothing later on.

Dip the paper strips into the flour mixture and place them onto the bag until it is thoroughly covered. Allow to dry. You may want to add a second coat. Once the head is ready, it is time to paint it. Be creative: purple pussycats, blue gorillas, pink ladies – anything goes. You can add hair made of yarn, sequined eyes – your choice. The doll can be dressed or used as a puppet.

Sock Doll

Take a large sock – man's or woman's, the bigger the better – and lay it flat. Cut off the cuff. Keeping it folded, cut the cuff in half. You have just prepared the arms. Sew up all the seams to the arms, leaving a hole to lace the stuffing in. Then finish closing the seams. Set the arms aside.

Take the rest of the sock and refold it so that the heel is underneath, and the part that was previously the edge is on top. The heel becomes the buttocks of the doll. Carefully cut into the cuff end up towards the heel, stopping about one and a half inches before the heel. You have just made two legs. Stuff the head (toe of the sock), using a rubber band to keep the head separate from the body. Stitch around each of the legs, leaving a hole for the stuffing. Stuff the body of the doll and the legs. Secure the hole.

Now stitch the arms onto the doll. Decorate and dress the doll any way you like. Buttons are good for eyes, as long as the doll is not for a child who is too young. For these children you can embroider the face, or even use indelible markers. The face will remain when the doll is washed.

Many of the children we treat who have physical and learning disorders have concomitant emotional problems that need to be addressed along with their primary disorders. And many children are referred with primary emotional problems. I used dolls to help them express their feelings as an excellent way to relieve the anxiety that prevent the children from progressing in therapy.

Using one's creative skills to produce a doll is one way that identity issues can be dealt with in a positive experience. Expressive play with dolls is a great way for children to voice their concerns through another entity without feeling compromised.

And grownups? Well, we're never too old for dolls!

The 'puzzle' behind the fun and fascination of activities

Originally published in *Advance for Occupational Therapy* March 17, 1997

The other day, wanting my students to experience an activity and its associated phenomena, I placed a jigsaw puzzle on the table in the student lounge and left. The next time I walked by, I noticed the outline of the puzzle was finished. Then I found several other puzzle boxes on the table, and the first one was back in the box. When I asked the students if they didn't like the first one, they laughed and said, no, they had simply taken it apart and put it together so many times that they decided to take out another one.

Where's Waldo I was followed by Where's Waldo II, and then by other puzzles that came through the door. Not only were the occupational therapy students working on puzzles – so were the physical therapy students! Everyone seemed to enjoy this low-pressure diversionary activity, especially as a break from studying for exams. And students who did not know one another were working together eagerly.

Later on, in class, we discussed the many things they had observed about how the puzzle itself structured their behavior and experiences.

When I was working in psychiatry, I always put a puzzle out on the table, and many times I used it to develop relationships with patients who were otherwise unwilling to communicate. I would just sit there, working on the puzzle. Soon someone would come over and join me. After a bit I would begin to ask them to sort colors and shapes. Pretty soon they were totally involved, and we would begin to talk about all manner of things.

Puzzle building is a compelling activity. It draws people to it of its own accord. There is something about those small, colorful pieces that demands they be placed together in an intelligible, complete form. In fact, there seems to be an inherent need for perceptual constancy that persists throughout life. Still, it is an activity that does not place pressure on those working on it. Everyone seems to recognize that they can work to their own purposes and extent.

The way one goes about doing a puzzle says a great deal. Some people look for all the edge pieces and construct a perimeter, while others take a more random approach. Some people sort the pieces by color and subject, working on their section apart from the whole. Still others work from the picture on the box, placing distinctive pieces where they are likely to fit when the puzzle is complete. Other people think that using the box as a guide is a violation of the 'rules', which of course they themselves have created.

Here you can see cooperation or not. Perceptual acuity or not. Persistence despite obstacles or not. Puzzles can be graded from simple to complex, both by the number of pieces and their sizes and shapes, for both children and adults.

Landscapes, artistic renditions and amusing arrays all come in various shapes and sizes, from miniature puzzles made for travel that can be finished up in minutes, or those with up to 1,000 or more pieces, that can take weeks to complete.

Right now, on the game table in my house, sits a 500-piece puzzle with a picture of medieval tapestry. My grandchildren and I are working on it together. We can do as much as we want and quit whenever we want, still feeling successful for as much as we've completed. Moreover, it is understood and expected that anyone else can come by and work on it as well. Everyone knows that jigsaw puzzles are like that.

Jigsaw puzzles are called that because they are made with a jigsaw. To make one, paste a poster or photograph to a piece of cardboard or wood, using a white glue such as Elmer's. Allow the picture board to dry thoroughly. Then turn the work upside down and trace curved lines on the reverse side, going up and down and side to side from edge to edge. Using a scroll or jigsaw with a fine blade, cut on the lines, being careful not to lose any of the pieces as they fall away. When you are finished cutting, put all the pieces into a bag until you are ready to work on the puzzle.

This is a project that several people can do, depending on their particular skills. Creating a personalized puzzle is not only good therapy – the finished product makes a great gift!

Saving the Environment

Last summer, the curator of our school's library gallery met up with one of our faculty. The curator needed something to place in the display window outside the gallery. Her window displays always attract a good deal of interest, so our faculty member suggested that we might be able to help with an interesting display. She referred the curator to me, since I had a class with a laboratory in which the students made some creative things that might be visually interesting in the window.

We arranged to meet at the occupational therapy laboratory to look around. As it happened, our class had just finished an exercise which I fondly call the 'trash project', so the room was filled with strange and interesting items.

The class is required to collect items they find and bring them into laboratory and dump them on the table. Everyone is then allowed to pick anything they want from the pile and make one or two projects from the items they find that have potential therapeutic purpose.

One group of students had assembled a long tube and a ball into a skinny and tall doll, complete with an apron made of a chair pillow and hair made of yellow yarn, topped with a hat made from a paper plate. She was very amusing and wound up as the centerpiece of the window display.

Another project was an old shoe box covered in bright fabric and a used washcloth bound in rubber bands, which was turned into a baby carriage pulled by a string. Two plastic milk jugs became a tossing game using masking tape wound into a ball. Empty soda bottles were filled with colored water and turned upside down to become a bowling game.

The curator was entranced and insisted on bringing the items over to the gallery to be displayed immediately, so we loaded up and off we went. My job was to write copy about how these items could be used therapeutically, which of course was the task the students had performed in class.

This display received lots of interest on campus, judging from the email messages we received. It gave us a good opportunity to highlight occupational therapy as a creative therapeutic (and thrifty) career.

Each year, my edict to the students is as follows: 'Now that you know how to run a therapy program without funds, I will haunt you if you ever let your management know you can do this. You need a budget!'

Following are some articles that explore the environment and issues of cost containment and recycling.

Hey, don't throw away all those six-pack rings yet!

Originally published in *Advance for Occupational Therapy* Oct. 16, 1995

It's easy to pick up a catalog and flip through it to find a selection of suitable crafts for the clinic. But it may be more meaningful – and more fun – to find things within the living environment. Not only is this approach economical, it supports the recycling effort being made nationwide today.

The community is a resource that often goes untapped. Combining the community trips in which many clinics engage with a hunt for supplies can imbue the trip with richer interest. It also can serve to illustrate cost-saving efforts.

Whether you go hunting in the city or the country, you can find many objects to construct creative projects that may be of value to both clients and their families. These things will differ according to where you live.

Interestingly shaped stones, for instance, can be polished and set into jewelry mounts, or used as touchstones, as Jane Sorensen described in her recent article on non-traditional practice ('Taking care of business', ADVANCE, Sept. 4).

Beachcombers find searching the sands relaxing and rewarding, and patients may also. Shells and driftwood found along the shore can be used to make many imaginative items. Vines of many kinds make good basket materials. Wild grape and honeysuckle are widely available and fun to collect.

The city is also a resource. My students each are required to bring in some kind of discarded plastic item. This mess of materials they describe as garbage goes into a pile on the lab table. Often included are Styrofoam™ packing popcorn, empty soda and milk cartons of all sizes, sheets of used plastic, small boxes previously used to store tubes of medications, coffee stirrers, film, film reels, used soap containers, broken lucite objects and fishing line.

Groups of students then set about constructing anything they decide to make using any of the available materials. The creativity they exhibit is astonishing. One group made an entire choo-choo train – including the engine, cars loaded with cargo, and a caboose. The medicine boxes were the cars; each car was attached to the other with a thread of plastic fishing line. Film reels served as the wheels. Brown coffee stirrers served as the cargo, looking for all the world like logs. Best of all, the students used the top of a liquid soap dispenser to represent a smokestack.

Other groups have made games from the objects they found. They tossed balls made of packing tape back and forth to be caught in cut-out milk bottles held upside down by the handles. They constructed board games of all kinds, as well as elaborate game strategies that made for great fun as teams participated in run-offs.

Artistry was not neglected. Sculptures appeared from all sorts of materials, some abstract and some representative. Masks, hats, vests, jewelry and toys emerged from the garbage heap.

You can develop these same kinds of activities in the clinic. In fact, the facility where you work may have items available that would make good materials for creative construction. Used X-ray film, while not as readily available as it once was, is sometimes still around. It can be used to make patterns, and even adaptive equipment such as a stocking pull-on device. In fact, the first one was actually made that way and was very functional.

Free materials from the world of man or nature abound. Their use is limited only by your imagination.

No budget: what do we do now?

Originally published in *Advance for Occupational Therapy* Sep. 21, 1998

A short while back I wrote a column titled, 'Where have all the trained OTs gone?' Among the several responses that I received was a letter from Mary McGee, a new occupational therapy assistant, who states that she is 'diligently trying to avoid pegs and cones for the simple fact that many patients do not see the reasoning behind these activities...' She went on to explain, 'Due to financial restraints and limited materials in our clinic, we have limited supplies on hand beside the basic occupational therapy tools, i.e. cones, pegs, Theraband, putty, etc. Perhaps you can guide me to a starting point in which I can begin to initiate different and new ideas to better motivate patients to reach their highest level of functioning.'

Well, before we talk about things, let's talk about thoughts. An occupational therapy department presents an image. Filling a department with artifacts that are meaningful develops a picture of what goes on in therapy. It may take some time to change the image of what is going on in this clinic, but changing an image results in different thinking. Once the thinking begins to change, it may be less difficult to convince funding sources of your needs.

Some of the answers may be within the control of the people who prepare department budgets and their ability to prepare budgetary arguments that are convincing. So let's think about what you've said.

First, you describe the 'basic occupational therapy tools' that are in the clinic as cones, pegs, Theraband, putty, etc. Are these supplies purchased from a commercial vendor of medical supplies? In my experience, supplies purchased from such vendors are more costly than those from other sources of occupational therapy materials. Comparative cost analysis can do wonders for obtaining budget approvals. The fact that patients will probably be better served by other materials also should contribute to the argument.

Second, not all materials have to cost money. Identifying donated sources of supply can be helpful. It may take some time to fill a department with meaningful tools. Start by using what you do have available.

I can remember my first job at Coney Island Hospital. The hospital and the department were just opening up at the time. Whoever had planned the department had ordered wonderful equipment and designed beautiful space in which to work, but no one had thought to order any supplies that we could use on the equipment. I can remember scavenging packing crates, and setting patients to the task of pulling nails out of the crates and hammering them flat. We also identified all our personal sources of supply.

My husband provided us with cans of printers' ink so we could get the hand cranked presses up and running. We identified a variety of sources in the community and wrote letters to them telling them about our needs. Many vendors were happy to provide us with their leftovers in exchange for a letter acknowledging their donations. We put notes up on bulletin boards, and were soon the recipients of fabric and other supplies. We scrounged nylon stockings from the nursing staff, and the patients cut them up and used them as stuffing for projects of various kinds.

All the projects they worked on were done for individualized therapeutic purposes, because the therapists were skilled in activity analysis and in grading activities, which included adapting environments, building projects and developing roles and relationships based on individual abilities. The patients felt they were doing things that were important, and contributing their efforts to the department as a whole was as important to them as making individual projects that were personally meaningful.

In my opinion, the reason occupational therapists became the splint makers is that they had all the materials at hand to create splints, and had the skill to manipulate these materials. Remember, early splints were made of metal, leather and other materials, used rivets, buckles and other such closures. Knowing how to make a pattern and transfer it to other materials was a skill every occupational therapist had from experience in crafting projects, and it was easily applied to splint-making.

By the way, do any of you remember the source of cones? They were originally the structures on which yarn is wound at the factory. These cones were in the occupational therapy clinics because they were left over after the looms were warped.

I believe occupational therapy practitioners have a professional responsibility to provide their patients with the tools needed to enhance their performance. If one is working in an environment where such tools are limited, the occupational therapy practice should not be limited because the environment is limited. Ultimately, the responsibility belongs to the occupational therapy practitioner, because he/she knows what is important to practice.

If you recognize that patients you are treating are not being treated appropriately, it is your responsibility to change things. If you do not make changes where changes are necessary, you are abdicating your own responsibility.

I believe that once you and your colleagues have decided to create an image of active occupation for your department, things will come to pass sooner than you imagine. When you stop restricting yourself by acknowledging your right to determine quality practice, all things are possible. Good luck!

The case for recycling 'stuff'

Originally published in *Advance for Occupational Therapy* June 15, 1998

In this volatile economic period, where the stock market goes up and down every day and every occupational therapy publication reports on managed care's effect on our income, it might be nice to think of money in other terms.

In a recent issue of *Countryside*, a homesteading magazine that I find time to read occasionally, I was reminded of how tangible materials keep their value. The article's premise was that if you save the old things, then you do not have to earn some cash you might otherwise need to buy new things with. Of course, homesteaders have refined this method to an art, because their survival depends on this skill. They are known to save everything from rubber bands to old socks, car parts and anything else they can get their hands on.

Now why does this behavior remind me of occupational therapists, particularly those of an age? All the years I was doing home health, the back end of my car looked like a veritable junkyard. I never knew when someone was going to need something, and with a little scavenging, I could pull out just the right piece of old wire, a special clamp, or a can of spray paint. For who knew what patients I would meet on any given day? And the clinic and the store were out of reach.

We women who did this often used to describe ourselves as 'bag ladies'. (The men did it too, but that epithet didn't quite apply to them.)

In all my years of practice, I have never turned down anyone's offer of 'stuff'. After all, you never know – I might need that stuff some day. Some of this stuff included leftover yarn from someone's sweater project, containers of every description, the rolls that are found inside toilet paper and paper towels, or the punched-out discards of a plastic manufacturer, that could be turned into sculptures.

What did we do with all this junk? I wish I could remember all the things that have found their way into my patients' homes. I remember, for example, that some of the old *Reader's Digest* magazines became Christmas angels. To do this you just fold each page back on itself so the book stands as a cone, spray paint it gold (or any other color that you like), and add a head and wings. Since so few activities require finger extension, this is a great way to enhance this motion, especially around the holidays. And if this is not the right time of year for angels, princesses make great children's toys any time of year.

There was always an old bench that needed refinishing, and there was always a patient for whom this activity was therapeutic. And the bench was really useful for positioning.

Stockings with runs in them made for the best stuffing in the world. Turning stockings into stuffing made a great project for someone practicing how to use scissors, never mind the various projects that needed the stuffing.

Socks – pairs or singles – are the greatest tools of all. Practicing removing a sock from one's hand, just by using one's finger movements, is a great strengthening exercise and can even become a game, working against the clock. And filling a sock with objects is good for stereognosis training. Turning socks into dolls is also great fun, so having a variety of different socks to choose from is great.

Needless to say, these projects were thrifty and they also required a bit of ingenuity.

I still find it difficult to purchase costly items from catalogs when a recycled alternative is available. I think one of the reasons that therapists got out of the habit of using recyclables is that it is often easier to obtain reimbursement for expensive items than it is to make the effort to obtain and store 'stuff'. Yet, by choosing to use standardized, manufactured items for therapy, a good bit of the humanity is removed from the therapeutic environment.

Items that are recycled have character. They bring with them a connection to the former owner, and they intimate control and creativity in which patients participate in their own recovery. And it makes delivering therapy so much more interesting for everyone, patient and therapist alike.

Putting out the challenge to find what's cost effective

Originally published in *Advance for Occupational Therapy* Oct. 21, 1996

I have a theory about health care economy, and here it is:

If a patient is returned to sustainable independent performance as a consequence of what has been done in therapy, that is cost containment. Saving money is assured by the effectiveness of what's purchased, not by the cost of the materials alone.

For many years I have wanted to test this theory – to do a study of the cost effectiveness of occupational therapy – but I never made it a priority and therefore never accomplished the goal. Unfortunately, I'm not alone. The few efficacy studies that have been done by occupational therapy have not focused on economic issues.

Occupational therapy is certainly a cost-effective service. When we enable patients to return to independent living, we cut costs for families, insurance companies and society as a whole. Yet we have not examined which of our treatments have the greatest cost effectiveness. My own view is that treatments which tend to engage patients and enhance their involvement in the effort will probably be most effective – and therefore, ultimately, cheapest.

So what does this mean in clinical terms? It means that you as a therapist must provide the most meaningful therapy for your patients or you will not be as effective as if you had.

You need special tools to provide meaningful therapy, but they are not expensive.

I am just old enough to remember that it never was easy to obtain supplies. At my first job at Coney Island Hospital, we took nails out of packing crates and had some patients hammer them straight, while others made projects from the crates themselves. Every therapist in the city had a note on the hospital bulletin board asking for used nylon hosiery which patients cut up into strips to stuff pillows and the like. Many of our sources for these materials were former patients and their families, who were all too pleased to contribute whatever they could to others to improve their health.

Therapy itself was often focused on making things for others, creating a meaningful endeavor with used scrap materials. The patients' satisfaction was enhanced by the appreciation expressed by the recipients and their families.

Making tangible objects is what crafts is all about. It permits patients to view and evaluate their own performance, and to gain the respect of others. It is far more meaningful to make a toy for a youngster with special needs than to put pegs in holes in meaningless rote fashion, contributing nothing to oneself or others in the process.

A good therapist should be able to construct a budget with a rationale that explains to purchasing officers the need for items. I rather suspect that the hesitation in ordering craft supplies springs from the therapist and not from management. Too many occupational therapists are unfamiliar with activity techniques and therefore are hesitant to order them for use in the clinic. Perhaps they are right. One should not order supplies for patients unless one is able to use them effectively.

Start at the beginning. Take an adult education course in the use of a craft. Learn how to use the tools correctly; that way you'll be able to teach others how. Periodically, try to have an in-service scheduled that incorporates the use of crafts. You might be surprised at the various skills your colleagues have and are willing to share.

Remember also that your students are resources. Many come to clinics with a background in activities they have learned in school or elsewhere. They need experience in teaching these to someone else. Gain your skills in all the ways you can. Then when it's time to do the budget next year, be sure to include the item you need.

If you are certain of its application in your setting, you can justify its purchase.

I'll bet your patients will get better faster. Will someone please do that research and get back to me?

Home, Garden and Beyond

The term context has entered the vocabulary of the profession in recent years. It is a welcome addition. For a time, it was accepted that occupational therapy was a medical profession, best delivered in hospitals and clinics, under the watchful eye of the physician whom the occupational therapist served as underling.

In the medical setting, there is a notion of precision that is pervasive. It is the same notion that leads scientific research. Careful standardization of procedures is called for. The problem with standardized procedures is that they are far from the ideas and procedures of ordinary living that are evident in people's lives.

When someone becomes disabled, the goal of occupational therapy is to return that person to meaningful living within the context of their former lives and roles. Inherent in that idea is that people lead unique lives.

Here is the dilemma as I see it: how can one return to a meaningful former life if one's therapy is restricted to standardized practices? Better the therapist should examine the context of a patient's life and utilize that context to deliver meaningful and restorative therapy. That is exactly what good therapists do. It is what young and inexperienced therapists would do too, if they knew they had the right and responsibility to do so.

The articles in this chapter are devoted to ideas about practice that extend beyond the traditional clinical environment ordinarily experienced in medical settings to the environments of home, garden, work and other meaningful places.

It is important to recognize that occupational therapy can be built around all activities, if one has a good understanding of the activities obtained through experience and activity analysis. That is one important thing about occupational therapy – it has to be experienced, both by therapist and by patient. To be a good therapist, one should be able to call upon a wide variety of activities, so one can draw upon them in practice, as appropriate.

These articles are designed to suggest some ideas for what is possible if you allow your notion of context to expand beyond the pages of a text to the world of experience. Your own experiences can undoubtedly initiate some other ideas. And most importantly, your patients can tell you what will work for them in their lives. They will be your best teachers.

Culture cooking makes for great occupational therapy

Originally published in *Advance for Occupational Therapy* Nov. 18, 1996

Cooking is a familiar activity among occupational therapists. We often have kitchens in our clinics, and having the equipment available seems to encourage us to use it in many ways. Many therapists find cooking to be a useful occupation, as a number of different kinds of patients can benefit from learning to prepare food.

Among the applications are learning to cook within the constraints of newly limiting physical disabilities (hand or shoulder injury, stroke, amputation); working in a group to enhance decision making skills and communication; engaging in familiar activities for patients with dementia; learning skills in self care for adolescents with a variety of disabilities; enhancing the ability to use memory in applied tasks, as is necessary for patients with post traumatic head injury.

To meet these goals, I frequently have seen therapists pull out packaged cake mixes, instant puddings or other prefabricated American food products for patients to cook up. Yes, instant products are very useful in that they often contain all the ingredients and utensils you will need. In addition, the directions on the boxes are explicit, and usually quite simple, allowing one to monitor patients' performance, or to encourage patients to do the job independently.

At the same time, I have sometimes wondered, 'Would I like to cook or eat these things?' You see, cooking to me is more visceral – more part of my cultural upbringing – so instant foods do not seem altogether appealing. I rarely use them at home and am more inclined to cook from natural ingredients. And I suspect that such is the case for many of our patients as well, especially older persons or those whose origins are in other lands, where instant foods are unavailable.

Cooking is part of everyone's culture. We are bound by the sights, smells and sounds of our heritages, as expressed in food. Because of the variety of cultures that contribute to our society, we have a wide number of resources available to us that can be used in the clinic.

Collecting recipes from many different cultures can become part of our professional experience. Selecting from them appropriately and adapting them to the needs of our clients should be among our professional skills.

Here are some food preparation experiences that were designed to meet patients' health and cultural needs.

One of my clients had a Colles fracture which healed very well, but because his arm had been immobilized in a sling for such a long time, he developed a debilitating shoulder weakness. Marc liked to cook, so he and I went into the kitchen and dragged out my chopping bowl and chopper, boiled the eggs, fried up the onions and liver, and he began to chop.

Making chopped liver is not difficult, it just requires persistence. Since he was a New Yorker by birth, he was motivated to chop until he thought it was just the right consistency. Not only was he pleased with the results, his family was delighted – Dad was cooking again.

A woman in a nursing home needed to increase her standing tolerance and balance following a hip fracture. Preparing the rugelach (rolled pastries) she usually made at home was just the right thing for her.

Using a rolling pin to stretch the dough allowed her to shift her balance while standing safely at the table. She sprinkled the dough with sugar, raisins, cinnamon – and love – before cutting the dough into triangles. She rolled each piece carefully and placed it on a cookie sheet, which was then put in the oven. She recognized that she was capable of performing this familiar task, and that was inordinately helpful in getting her to realize that she would be capable of returning home.

Sometimes one can simply open up a few cans and come up with a simple and delicious dish. Mixed-bean salads are found in many different cultures and differ according to the variety of beans and the spices used. So Moroccan, Indian, Mexican and vegetarian cuisines can be made from very plain ingredients. Chances are, your patients can tell you exactly what ingredients are best.

Shopping for food can meet many needs as well. The most memorable shopping adventure I went on with a patient was with a young man with concentration problems. He would be discharged soon from a psychiatric hospital to live alone in an apartment. His inability to make decisions easily was most apparent in the supermarket, particularly when it came to choosing eggs. Brown or white? Large or small? Commercial or free range? Expensive or cheap? It was all a great muddle to him.

We developed some strategies that he could use to help him get through the process, and he was able to use them successfully to reduce his anxiety.

Food has healing qualities, both for what it does for us internally, and for what it can offer in terms of its occupational opportunities. When food preparation is combined with its cultural qualities, it is more apt to meet clients' needs. Try it, you may like it. I know your patients will!

Fall: it's finally in the air

Originally published in *Advance for Occupational Therapy* Sep. 25, 2000

School buses are on the move. Sounds of football and soccer are heard in the schoolyards. Nights are getting cool, and it's almost time to bring in the harvest.

And as the leaves in the Northeast turn to red and orange and yellow, and flutter to the ground, they bring with them many ideas for activities for people of all ages and with all levels of performance capacity.

Collecting leaves is a great activity. Aside from the bending and reaching that are needed, there are sorting tasks available. Large, small; red, yellow, green; maple, oak and elm. How to use these leaves in artistic projects challenges the creativity of therapists and patients alike. Placemats, wall hangings and book covers make fun projects. Leaves also make good stencil shapes that can be applied to furniture as well as walls.

The gardens we planted in the spring and summer are coming ripe now. Tomatoes are abundant and ready for picking. Not only are they great for eating fresh, but making sauce is an ideal group activity. Peeling and slicing vegetables such as peppers and onions to add to the tomatoes requires fine-motor action. And the rewards are great – a festive meal in which everyone who participates builds confidence and self-image. Especially if the meal is prepared for important guests – read that as parents, spouses, siblings, children, teachers, volunteers, therapists, etc.

Going out to pick apples is another wonderful fall activity that requires reaching. One can make a sack that hangs from the shoulder to place the apples in, making their carrying easier. And making applesauce from the pickings is great fun as well. Apples are washed, boiled, and riced, requiring bilateral strength and coordination. The aroma they produce is stimulating and satisfying. Cooking in the occupational therapy department is a great way to attract attention from one's colleagues, especially if one is able to share the product.

Off now to pick the pumpkins. Selecting one's favorite shape may require a trek through a pumpkin field. Many farms in the countryside let groups come to pick in the fields. Maybe the person in the wheelchair can hold the pickings for those who are unable to carry the heavy pumpkins themselves. Carefully assigning jobs so that the entire group participates and each feels an important member is how the occupational therapy practitioner can effectively coordinate the trip.

How about an old-fashioned hayride? For youngsters it may be a new experience. For oldsters, it may stimulate memories of times gone by. Getting out into the community to smell the wonderful scent of mown hay is a worthwhile trip. (Just remember, some people are allergic to hay. As with all events, make sure that all the participants' health needs are being met.) And be sure to obtain the appropriate permissions.

Just getting a group together to reminisce about the fall can be a therapeutic experience for people who are shut in. What does the fall mean to you? And what does it mean to your clients? If you try, you can make this fall a memorable event for them.

Water, water, everywhere, so have some fun

Originally published in *Advance for Occupational Therapy* July 23, 2001

When summer comes, I can't help but think of water. I think of children as they play in the sprinkler or sit in an inflated pool. I think of the swimming pool and waves on the shore, surfboarding and playing in the sand. I think of playing in rivers and lakes while kayaking, canoeing or water skiing.

All of these activities are ordinarily part of the experiences of the general public, but only recently are they becoming an expectation of people with disabilities. Moreover, many of these activities have potential therapeutic application, with a little creative ingenuity.

Playing dodge ball under the sprinkler is a great equalizer for people in or out of wheelchairs. Everyone, of all ages, can move about, get wet, and have fun while being refreshed. Learning to swim is a milestone event, a suitable challenge for people of all ages. There are races of all sorts to organize. One can race using standard swimming strokes measured by speed, or one can set up a variety of other swim events. Competitions between teams include games in which objects are carried across the pool, or endurance itself is the goal. Just learning to float on a board in a swimming pool can be a lot of fun. Having a lift available can make this an accessible activity for everyone.

If swimming isn't your cup of tea, try water exercising. Since water is resistive but buoyant, it makes a good exercise medium that has become very popular. There are lots of water toys available to make moving in the water a fun experience – paddleboards and noodles, rings and weights. Pool exercise can be a good socializing event, perfect for group building.

People with disabilities of various sorts join clubs in which they can participate in modified surfing activities. Surfing does not have to be the standing sport like we see in the movies. There are 'boogie boards' designed to use in prone position. There is even adapted water skiing for people with disabilities. It's hard to think of water skiing as a sit-down event, but special seating has been developed for this active sport to make it possible for many different people to actively participate. For example, blind individuals compete accompanied by a sighted companion.

Remember: water sports do not require being in the water. Boating is a great opportunity to enjoy the great outdoors. Whether you prefer sailing or motor boating, there are lots of ways to participate. Sculling, otherwise know as crew, is a rowing activity that has been adapted to enable people with balance problems and paralysis to participate via special harnesses and seating. Competition or cooperation can be the focus, since crew can be an individual or team sport.

Expanding opportunities for water participation requires attention to water safety. Be sure and do the right things! Take a water or boating safety course. Arrange to have a lifeguard in attendance. Follow the rules of the pool. At my house it is no jumping or diving. Use the appropriate sunscreen. And enjoy the rest of the summer.

There's no end to what you can do with summer plants

Originally published in *Advance for Occupational Therapy* May 20, 1996

Gardening, on a big or small scale, is an excellent activity for nearly everyone. From youngest to oldest, the use of seeds and plants can be exciting, stimulating and the expression of participation in the magic of nature. Going back to playing in the dirt is a wonderful reminiscence of childhood. The memories that gardens can elicit are very special.

Many years ago I was a student working in a tuberculosis sanitarium, just before the advent of effective TB drugs closed such centers. One activity the patients enjoyed was to construct terreria. As part of our student projects, we went out shopping during our lunch break to find small succulent plants and appropriate planters to make dish gardens. The more active patients put these gardens together, and the bed-bound patients found a great deal of pleasure in watching the plants thrive.

Children love to watch seeds erupt and grow into plants. One quick, fun garden is to plant a dish with grass seed. It needs to be kept moist until it sprouts. It can even be 'mowed' using small scissors. You can cut the grass to various heights, creating a design in the 'lawn'.

Some flower seeds, like marigolds, are quick sprouting and make a colorful display. Marigolds come in many varieties. The flowers can be sprouted in paper cups or seedling pots, and then transplanted to an outdoor area. Keep it well watered until the plant adjusts to its new home.

Bulbs also produce beautiful dish gardens. Hyacinths, tulips and daffodils can be forced, but the plant with which you will have the most success is paper white narcissus. And it offers a lovely aroma when it blooms. Bulbs need to spend some time in the freezer first, to make them think that they have experienced a cold winter underground. Once removed from the cold they can be placed in a glass tray over some gravel or stone. Set the bulbs so the points are up and the rootlets down. Push them into the gravel bed so they stand touching each other. About six to a dish makes a nice display. The dish should be filled with enough water to cover the bottom quarter inch of the bulbs. The water evaporates quickly especially in a heated room, so be sure to refill the dish every day. Pretty soon, the roots will begin to grow out among the stones, and the bulbs will erupt with long, green stalks that look like onions. Wait a little longer and the flowers will appear. The project is easy to do and quick enough to show a change over a short period of time.

The outdoor garden is the best of all. Not everyone has the luxury of sufficient space for a clinic garden, but if it is at all possible, it offers so many therapeutic opportunities: resistive activities, cooperative tasks, planning and myriad other opportunities.

A raised garden is particularly useful, as it allows one to be able to engage in gardening from a wheelchair. My nursing home patients taught me about gardening. Did you know that tomatoes can be picked and frozen whole? Place them on a sheet in a freezer, then put them in a plastic bag. When you need tomatoes for cooking, pull one or more out, run them under water and the skins will slip off, making the tomato ready for use in stews, soups, sauces or whatever.

So flowers are not the only things to plant. There is nothing quite so pride-inducing as harvesting one's own produce and sharing it with others. Lots of vegetables are quick growing and fun to grow. Lettuce, an early summer crop, can be harvested in its seedling form. Spread the seeds on the raked earth, covering them lightly with soil. When they sprout, just pull out the crowded plants to thin them out, snip off the roots and eat the young lettuce. The taste is delightful, and the vegetables can be added to any salad.

Radishes are also quick growing and early. Tomatoes are everyone's favorite and can be grown in pots. They take a little longer to come to ripeness but are fun to watch as the flowers emerge and turn into fruit. Of course, if you have room there are the vines of cucumbers, squash and pumpkin. Zucchini and summer squash are endless bearers.

The project doesn't end in the garden. It continues on into the kitchen, and we all know how useful that is as a therapeutic environment. (Like apples for applesauce as we near the fall and prepare to shut the garden down and stick with indoor plants like philodendron and aloe, that can give us pleasure in the cold months.)

The therapeutic applications of these activities are endless.

One needs only to know how to garden to be able to analyze the possibilities.

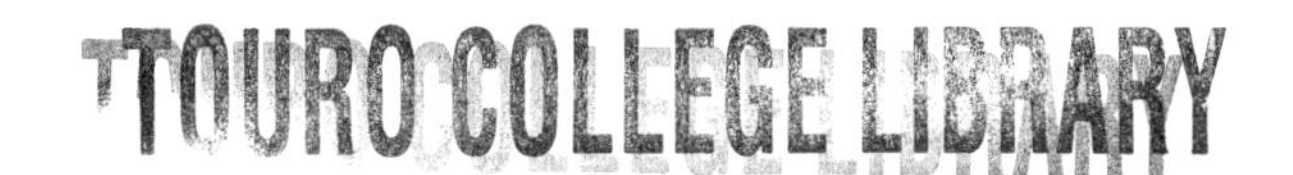

Planting the seeds of accessible activity

Originally published in *Advance for Occupational Therapy* July 26, 1999

Now that the warm weather has come, I'm back in the garden again. I have planted my seeds, hoed the rows, plucked the weeds, and seen some success.

The peas are up, the broccoli is full and leafy, the tomato plants are full of flowers, and the pepper plants and eggplant are coming along, too. The lettuce is the leafiest I have every produced. And our dinners are delicious as we take advantage of the seasonal produce. From planning to planting to harvesting to consuming and sharing, gardening is meaningful in my life.

Best of all, this year I don't have to bend to tend the vegetables I planted. During the cool weather months, we built some raised garden boxes, and they are really working out well. These garden boxes have made planting and weeding so easy that I don't know why everyone isn't gardening this way. Next year we are going to build some more.

When we decided to build the garden boxes the primary criterion we used was that they had to be wheelchair accessible. You see, I'm planning ahead for the time when anyone in the family needs to use a wheelchair. It would be terrible to love to garden and not be able to do so because it is an inaccessible activity.

We made sure that the garden boxes were at the right height, wide enough that someone can reach to the center easily from a seated position, and positioned so that a wheelchair could fit between the boxes. Specifically, they are approximately two and a half feet high, three feet across and eight feet long. The boxes are built side by side along the long dimension, with a three-and-a-half-foot-wide path between them. Right now the boxes are surrounded by straw, but the area can easily be converted to a firmer surface for a wheelchair to move upon, should that become necessary.

The garden is not the only area in our home that now takes wheelchair access into consideration. All the construction around here in the last few years has considered accessibility. When we built an outside brick staircase to reach a raised backyard garden area, we left an access route for a wheelchair that considers the grade. We haven't built the path yet. It is still a soil-filled area, but it will be very easy to cement should that become necessary.

Planning for accessibility is very important. I learned this personally when my father required the use of a wheelchair. Unfortunately, our property is built on a hill and is not readily convenient for wheelchair use.

It is much easier to keep accessibility in mind when you are building a home from scratch. It requires a bit more ingenuity when you are renovating a home and grounds, but the fruits of your efforts are worth it.

Sometimes we tend to think about 'accessibility' as being specialized equipment or carpentered construction, but I think about it fundamentally as a means for doing.

It's necessary to enable people to engage in the many different types of activities that are part of their lives. Active occupation is the driving principle that governs accessibility.

It is important to understand the lifestyle of the person who requires access tools. Disability comes in many forms, and therefore it may offer many different kinds of restrictions.

Merging one's knowledge of dysfunction with one's knowledge of patients' interests is vital. For example, exterior terrain is a significant problem for individuals with postural uncertainty associated with degenerative disorders that cause knee and back problems. Unstable terrain prevents them from participating in activities that have meaning in their lives.

Because enjoying the outdoors is so important to my own life, accessible gardening is a must. Building the boxes is easier for two people without disability than it would be for one person with disability. So morbidity is put aside to plan for a future that will allow for favorite activities and meaningful living, regardless of changes in circumstance.

What are your favorite activities? Are they possible for you should life alter your circumstances? Do you have to start thinking now how you will perform later down the road?

While we do not often plan this way for our own lives, this is exactly what we must do for our patients' lives. Recognizing the need to plan ahead for ourselves will deepen an understanding of the meaning of the active occupation in which we engage. Thinking that way for ourselves will tend to make us better at thinking that way for our patients.

And isn't that our job?

There's lots of things to do 'lookin' out my back door'

Originally published in *Advance for Occupational Therapy* July 17, 1995

I have the good fortune to live on a small farm in western New Jersey. Its broad pastures, animals, trees, gardens and swimming pool have provided me lots of opportunities for treating patients. Some of the activities I use here are easily done indoors, but the most interesting ones are those that only can be done outside.

Occupational therapy used to be disparagingly described as 'basket weaving', as if this were meaningless. Yet pulling the honeysuckle vines out of a pine tree and sitting on the hill creating a basket was both gratifying and strengthening for a patient recovering from a Colles fracture and diminished strength in the shoulder secondary to the prolonged use of a cast and sling. For her, making a basket from nature was great fun as well as therapeutic. The finished product became a reminder of her recovery as well as a souvenir of some beautiful days in the country.

A group of children with special needs came to the farm to celebrate the end of the school year. Together, each of them learned to fold a sheet of paper into a small boat. They decorated their boats with watercolor paints, expressing themselves through their designs. After the boats were painted, the children lay down at the edge of the pool and placed their boats in the water. At the sound of a bell, the children let their boats go, and blew on them, stirring the water to encourage them to float away to the opposite side of the pool. When the race was over, it was time for dessert and a dip in the pool.

Two brothers with learning disabilities went outdoors to play blindfold games. Each one in turn hid items in the grass and gave his brother directions for finding the items. Right, left, over the barrel, inside the box, under the bar. Then find the fragrant flowers and collect five smooth pebbles. And for a special treat, let's feed the goats.

Picking fruit is another activity that extends beyond the orchard. Reaching up to pick the apples, and bending over to put them into a basket is good exercise, much more satisfying than a repetitious exercise regimen. Then to the kitchen to cook the apples in their skins, and into the ricer for applesauce, a good low-calorie dessert.

Actually, the vegetable garden at the psychiatric unit of the hospital where I once worked was a favorite of my patients – as well as the nursing staff. Every morning in the spring and summer when the weather was suitable, the group went out to dig, plant, hoe, mulch, fertilize, pick, and carry their harvest into the kitchen to add to lunch. The patients did not know how hard it had been initially to convince administration that the lawn behind the hospital should be dug up for that garden.

Mixing cement for the path beside the outdoor railroad garden is easily done with a tub, a hoe, some water and a pre-cast form. An adolescent recovering from head injuries that needed repetitive resistive physical activity and quick gratification enjoyed this job. The outdoor railroad offers so many different opportunities for activities that a group could easily work together on several components at the same time.

Digging a pond and laying out a miniature river bank and waterfall is fun and creative. Wiring electrical connections requires concentration and dexterity.

Using the environment to its fullest offers many opportunities for meaningful activities. I'm sure that your own outdoor environment can offer many new ideas, making therapy interesting and refreshing for you as well as your patients.

Considering public education and the kitchen cabinet

Originally published in *Advance for Occupational Therapy* Jan. 20, 1997

After 25 years of living in the same home and having watched its various parts fall away and the appliances die of old age, we decided to redo the kitchen. Consequently, I have been watching two men installing the new cabinetry.

One is clearly very experienced and uses his tools and know-how very efficiently. The other bumbles around – is not sure of the names of the tools, or which one is best for which part of the job. He is an apprentice and is learning by doing, and by the feedback he gets from his work and his supervisor.

While the less experienced man is younger, he is not so young that one would not think he might be more adept at tool use by now. But one also might wonder why he should be. What opportunities has he had to learn how to use tools?

Today's schools offer few opportunities to learn how to use tools and make objects with them. Somehow, we seem to think people learn best by learning abstractly at the outset. We save tangible learning for later, if at all. As a result, many young people are all thumbs when it comes to making objects and using tools. They are delayed in learning manipulative skills.

Standards for learning set within the educational system serve as the foundations for learning for special children. And so we spend huge amounts of time teaching them to hold a pencil and write, so that education can proceed. Only in the high school years does the system begin to recognize that a work role lies ahead, and this child is probably not going to do a job that requires the use of a pencil.

John Dewey, the famous American educator and philosopher who was responsible for the concept of 'learning by doing', recognized that engaging in activity contributed to learning, and in fact, served as its very foundation. The activities he chose for his educational program were tangible, and they were grounded in social needs and practices based on the history of society.

Dewey assumed that groups working together on projects could contribute to their own and others' learning when the activities allowed them to function together to their mutual benefit. Together his students learned to create objects that would allow their group to function actively, and in doing so, they learned the skill they needed to do the jobs.

From the earliest grades students engaged in constructive activities – gross and fine motor – that built their physical, intellectual and social skills. Each semester they learned a new set of skills, paralleling the activities in which various earlier societies had engaged. One year they imitated tasks of Native Americans such as clay work, basketry, and leatherwork, not only learning how these activities were done, but how they were instrumental in helping everyone in the group to survive.

The next year, students learned tasks that were developed later in history, such as carpentry and farming. And again, as they learned the skills, they also learned the contributions these activities offered to the betterment of all. For example, in order to be able to do carpentry, one needs to be able to read a ruler accurately, or the job will come out incorrect. So as students learned how to measure and calculate angles, their math skills grew along with their dexterity. From the active occupations in which they engaged, their learning increased, enabling them to proceed still further.

It seems to me that Dewey had the right idea. Active occupation (a term Dewey originated and discussed in 1916, a year before the first occupational therapy association was founded) is a means of learning. The integration of mind and body in active occupation is a principle of occupational therapy and the foundation on which our practice should rest.

By analyzing which skills one needs to have in order to be a contributing member of society, one can structure and adapt a graded activity program that will lead to the development of the needed skills. That is, the focus must be: what will this individual be able to do to contribute to society to his or her greatest level? (Such contribution would create not only personal satisfaction but positive feedback from the society.) And, what does this person need to learn to do so he or she can meet those goals?

Developmentally delayed youngsters take longer to learn skills than do other children. So delaying the onset of certain kinds of experiential learning to the later years of school may be the wrong route to take. Learning activities early that can translate into work roles in later years may be a more valuable approach in education. Moreover, mastering those tasks may contribute to learning. That's what Dewey thought.

I wonder: Would that inept carpenter's assistant be more skilled if he had learned to wield a hammer and screwdriver in pre-school? And I'll bet his behavior would have been better, too, because the energy he expended would have made him more willing to sit at his desk when those writing skills came up.

Bread: it can be the staff of your staff's life in the clinic

Originally published in *Advance for Occupational Therapy* Feb. 17, 1997

Looking for a modality you can use with kids, older adults, hand patients, stroke patients and many others as well? Try a loaf of bread.

For those of you who think bread-making is impossible without a bread machine, here's a recipe I have used many times for many purposes, and shared with many people over the years:

1 package of yeast
3/4 cup of water
1 teaspoon sugar
1 egg
1 stick of soft margarine
a pinch of salt
4–5 cups of flour

Combine the yeast and 1/4 cup of the water. Sprinkle the sugar over the yeast mixture and set it aside for 10 minutes, to activate. Place $3^1/2$ cups of flour in a large bowl. Break the egg into the flour; add the margarine, salt and yeast mixture, and mix ingredients thoroughly by hand.

If the mixture is too dry, add water gradually. When the mixture begins to feel like dough, but sticky, turn it out onto a well floured surface and knead. Press with the heels of the hands into the mixture, lifting and turning the dough and adding flour as you work.

When the dough is smooth, place in a clean bowl that has been lightly oiled, turning the dough over so the top becomes the bottom, and both surfaces are lightly oiled.

Cover with a clean towel, and set aside to rise in a warm place. When the dough has risen, punch it down and let it rise again. After it has risen again, divide the dough into three parts, and form them into rounds. Place on a greased baking sheet, cover and allow to rise again.

Bake for approximately 35–40 minutes at 350 degrees F. The surface should be golden brown, and should thump if you tap it. This recipe can be enhanced by adding raisins, caraway or anything delectable that you choose. It tolerates inexperienced hands, but try it once before you use it with patients because kneading is an acquired skill.

Of course my family has enjoyed this bread whenever I have decided to bake it over the years, but I have also found it useful for many different kinds of individual and group activities. Baking has universal appeal.

In a children's group, I assigned each of the children the job of bringing in one of the ingredients as an exercise in remembering. (Of course, I had backups as needed.) After washing their hands, the children combined the ingredients, kneaded the dough and put it aside to rise. I had brought with me another dough I had prepared at home previously and kept refrigerated. When I arrived, I set that dough in a warm place to rise as we worked. This way we were able to continue to make the loaves, put the bread into the oven to bake, and have it ready when the children left.

Each child brought home an aromatic loaf he had prepared and braided himself for his family to enjoy. To make a braided loaf, just divide the almost-ready-to-bake dough into three sections and roll each into a 'snake'. Place the three snakes together at on end and braid the sections together. Tuck the ends in underneath and set on a baking sheet to rise.

In a nursing home, nothing works better than bread for bringing people together. This recipe and others (for cookies, etc.) have enticed even the most reluctant patients into the activity room. The smell of baking bread is an unrivaled drawing card. Schedule the baking session just before the residents' annual fair or sale, and there is another appealing item for customers to purchase. Residents derive a great deal of satisfaction from that.

My hand patients have also baked bread. Bread dough is more satisfying than theraputty. The best part of this recipe is that one can do it in stages so there is time to do other tasks or to rest. The dough needs to rise several times, but it can be kept in the refrigerator overnight between risings without impairing its flavor. The baker can start the task one day and finish it the next.

Nothing is more effective as a socialization tool than a loaf of bread. It's ideal for the psychiatric clinic. The smell and taste bring back memories as the dish is being passed around. Add a little jelly – and maybe even some peanut butter –and you have a meal that's a warm reminder of childhood.

The ability to sequence while following a recipe, the need to keep track of time and measurements, the strengthening of hands, the opportunities of cooperation with others, and the sensory feedback one derives from this activity are priceless. Touching, seeing and smelling one's success and hearing the comments from others who have the opportunity to smell and taste the product, all contribute to the therapeutic experience.

When you bake in the occupational therapy department, the aromas drift down the halls to neighboring departments, attracting all manner of folk. Hungry residents, nurses on break, maintenance personnel and lots of other people become occupational therapy's best friends by following their noses.

If you try this, let me know how the bread came out, and what kinds of responses you got.

The key to self-worth may be right at your fingertips

Originally published in *Advance for Occupational Therapy* Oct. 19, 1998

The other day my granddaughter Alex and I were discussing our nails. (It's the sort of thing grandchildren and grandparents do when we are not discussing the common enemy: their parent, our child...)

Anyway, while her nails looked great, I bemoaned the fact that my manicure was ruined and I needed to redo it. Alex is an expert at these things at the tender age of 10. 'Gram-cracker,' she responded, calling me that to get my attention, 'did you put on a base coat? And did you apply two coats of polish? And then did you put on a top coat?'

I told her no, I hadn't done most of those things, but that my love of the garden had ruined my manicure because I never think about putting on gloves until it's too late.

But then I began to think. Clearly, this child knew more about nail care than I did, and I really needed to bring my knowledge base up to the modern era. I had heard people talking about French manicures, tips, acrylics, paste-ons – and I had no real certainty about which was what.

I had seen all kinds of decorative designs on other people's nails. There were stripes and dots, and symbols of various holidays in every color imaginable. It all seemed like lots of fun, but I was grossly uninformed about the details.

So I made an investment in my education – I hot-footed it off to the nearest manicurist for a professional job. And by golly, Alex was right. Base coat, two layers of color and a top coat came along with a hand massage with oil and a drying period in a heated, cage-like device. I learned about tips and other artificial additives that could be purchased to make one's nails look spectacular. And I realized that one should always keep up with the latest in grooming, especially if one is an occupational therapist.

In every clinical practice in which I have ever participated, patients loved to have their hands manicured. I've done it with psychiatric patients, stroke patients, school children and home health patients. And I now notice that it is one of the ways in which students love to 'play' when the stress of classroom demands becomes too great.

Paying attention to one's nails is a relaxing occupation for many people, whether they are doing it themselves or having someone else do it. From the selection of the polish to the grooming of the nails themselves, there comes a feeling of self-expression and self-caring. One's hands are an intimate expression of self and doing. They tell others about you, and are a good place to start when teaching patients the skills they must develop to care for themselves.

In a psychiatric clinic, the value of grooming groups is well documented. These groups orient patients to themselves and others around them. Beyond issues of self-worth, a manicure can help patients resolve finger agnosia and apraxia. Without certainty regarding finger agnosia, astereognosis is bound to occur. In fact, finger agnosia may be the cause of it. Helping patients differentiate their fingers from one another can be a first step in resolving this spatial disorder.

Embedding finger gnosis exercises in the manicuring process is a natural and healthful approach to this treatment, and it is relevant for children as well as adults. Handwriting difficulties that many children we see exhibit can be attributed to misidentification of fingers and finger movements. Using nail polish in creative ways, therapists can teach youngsters to identify their fingers correctly, and improve movement patterns and writing skills.

Use games that incorporate identifying nail polish markers. These techniques are similar to those games we teach kids to help them learn to identify body parts: 'Head, shoulders, knees and toes, knees and toes..., etc.' 'This little piggy went to market' is one of the finger or toe games, but it is too juvenile for older children or adults.

Hand therapists also may find manicures helpful in aiding patients who must deal with changed body images. The hands are a very personal and visible part of the body. The attention to fingers and nails that a manicure offers can help one accept this new image. And of course when one does the manicure herself, she is practicing fine-motor skills.

If you play with your food, do it right

Originally published in *Advance for Occupational Therapy* Feb. 22, 1999
By Isaac S. Friedman (one of Dr Breines' students, as guest author in her column)

'Don't play with your food!'

How many generations of kids have heard that? Of course, it means 'now it's time to eat, so don't dawdle, don't procrastinate and don't be disrespectful'. But author J. Eiffers has another idea. *Play with Your Food*, he says, in his 1997 book by that title (Stewart, Tabori and Chang, New York).

Eiffers believes food – especially fruits and vegetables – is 'playful' in its own right. (Have you ever found an odd-looking vegetable that looks like a funny face, a cute animal, a contorted body, a mini-monster or an overgrown insect?)

Fruits and vegetables seem to invent their own visual puns, he says. Remember when Mr Potato Head used real potatoes?

Indeed, food decoration is actually an art in fine restaurants and amid caterers as well as on the decks of cruise ships. But occupational therapists can use it to increase interest in cooking activities or entertain youngsters in therapy. The creative aspect of food decoration is a psychosocial link to your patients' inner thoughts and feelings.

The goal of this activity is to produce new images suggested by the fruits and vegetables themselves, with an absolute minimum of alteration: a slit here for the mouth, two slices there for the raised ears, two holes for the eyes, etc. If the original piece has a stem sticking out, use it as a tongue or a nose. If there is a root cluster, like that on an onion or leek, use it as hair or a beard. The idea is to make a whole new animal, face or object, as far as possible, out of the existing features of the regular piece.

Eyes can be the indicators of emotion, personality and mood. A variety of fruits and veggies, from beans to grapes to olives, make great eyes. Whatever works for you is valid. In some cases, simple slits with a knife are enough to indicate eyes, and there would be no need to introduce separate elements. In other cases, certain animals or faces may not have eyes at all, but just depressions in the skin of the food that might suggest eyes.

It is important to look at all possibilities for placing the eyes, because the starting point is usually the nose, and you work outward from there. Move your beans or grapes or olives around the 'face' to see the different opportunities. Note how the personality of your creation changes as you shift the eyes around – wider apart, closer together, higher, lower, and so on.

Anything that sticks out of the fruit or vegetable is a potential nose. Noses tend to be natural rather than created from carving or added elements. Once you identify the nose, other features will fall into place. Be sure to rotate the piece and look at every angle to find the best position for the nose.

Ears! They can be cut and folded or added as separate pieces. To make fold-out ears, outline their shape with your knife, leaving a fairly large area of attachment at the base.

Carefully slice beneath the skin and gently roll the ear out from tip to base. Patient and gradual rolling will prevent the ear from tearing. For very large ears, do not be afraid to cut far back on the fruit or vegetable.

With leafy veggies, you can just fold the leaves out to make ears. When you add them as separate pieces, you can cut and shape them from any desired food, not just the one you were starting from. Again, once you have fashioned add-on ears move them all around the larger piece to see where they best belong. When you have found the right spots, make the appropriate slots with your knife and insert the ears.

Mouths can be found (natural) or made (carved). In some cases they may be minimal, and in others not necessary at all. If you do carve a mouth, start small. You can always make it bigger. Teeth can be either carved or added (rice, corn kernels, almonds, etc.) Make the holes and then press them in.

For carving more complicated objects such as baskets, flowers, etc., you need to look at a picture and kind of trace it onto the fruit. This requires a lot of hand maneuvering, so be careful not to cut yourself or overcut the fruit or vegetable.

Here's a list of animals/objects I have carved into fruits/vegetables, along with the items needed.

- Basket – watermelon or cantaloupe
- Flowers – radish, cucumber
- Angry face – navel orange, black-eyed peas
- Hawaiian lady – artichoke, mushroom, food coloring
- Teddy bear – brown peach, black peas
- Mouse – brown peach, cloves
- Octopus – banana, black-eyed peas
- Palm tree – pineapple
- Bunny rabbit – green pepper, snow peas, almonds
- Pig – lemon, food coloring

Yes, Virginia, there is activity-based occupational therapy

Originally published in *Advance for Occupational Therapy* Oct. 20, 1997

There actually are some therapists out there who use activities in practice! And I believe it because I've seen it with my own eyes.

Recently, through e-mail correspondence about an article I had written, I received a wonderful invitation to visit the Menorah Park Home for the Aging near Cleveland, Ohio. Here, Ruth Plautz, OTR, is the director of rehabilitation services, and Mary Rinas, OTR, is director of occupational therapy. These two creative occupational therapists head a rehab program that makes activity a central theme for the residents and staff of this exemplary facility.

Along with the customary yet artistic table tasks which are displayed throughout the facility, I saw the life of a community incorporated into the life of the home. In fact, it was hard to remember that this was primarily a nursing home. Once I even had to ask, 'Where are the beds?', because the residents were so actively engaged.

The horticulture center was manned by head injured patients when I visited. They raised unusual plants to sell in the gift shop. The industry was evident; the plants flourished, along with the patients.

I was surprised to see the handsomely accoutered room that housed a bank and post office, making a Main Street to visit for business activities. Provided with that opportunity, residents have the means to govern their own affairs, in privacy and with self-respect.

The animal center was filled with beautiful finches, a great fluffy gray rabbit and several other warm and fuzzy creatures. I found it hard to leave the area to continue my tour, but there were more delights down the road. The puppy-in-residence in the dementia unit was happy to receive attention from everyone – residents, staff and visitors.

Best of all was the marvelous child day care center, which gave residents a chance to watch children play as they visited with family members. Day care personnel take the children around the home to visit residents who are unable to get around on their own. What joy these youngsters give to these surrogate grandparents. And the attention provided to the youngsters, whose parents are at work, could not be better.

Indoor and outdoor play areas and gardens encouraged intergenerational activity and therapy in many ways. Parallel bars sat side by side with swings and gliders, providing therapy tools in a delightful environment that seemed more a sculpture garden than a pain-for-gain sweat shop.

The chapel was as beautiful as any religious center in the community. It was designed with accessible ramping to allow wheelchair-users and ambulatory residents to attend services in comfort and serenity. Services were also transmitted by audio and video to those unable to get out.

The gardens everywhere are cared for by residents and volunteers, and look professionally manicured. Several areas throughout the home have raised garden beds built so that they can be managed from wheelchairs. And many of the gardens had vegetables growing among the flowers, allowing the residents to raise crops to harvest and eat.

Cooking and baking areas are found throughout Menorah Park so that residents can prepare their favorite recipes and celebrate their holidays throughout the gustatory calendar.

Residents who want to work are enrolled in a sheltered workshop complete with a timeclock on which they punch in and out. This cadre of dedicated workers fulfills contracts with outside manufacturers. Computers were set up in this area to encourage e-mail visits to and from grandchildren.

When my hosts asked me how to improve their activity programming, I began to laugh. I had never before seen a place as well equipped and well planned as this one. Who was I to tell them what to do? I was here to learn.

As you can see, activity was everywhere. It was the heart of the home and the heart of the occupational therapy program. Everyone valued it, and everyone was invested in it.

With an environment of this scope, occupational therapy can be delivered creatively, meaningfully and efficaciously.

Bravo, Menorah Park!

The therapy that's in your office

Originally published in *Advance for Occupational Therapy* March 16, 1998

Having recently experienced a change in personnel in my office, I began to think of the myriad tasks one has to learn in order to make the office function optimally. That led me to think about how I have often used many of these same tasks as therapy in various settings. I'm sure if you looked around your office, you, too, would find a number of activities that would be suitable for therapeutic skill building.

I keep a special 5-inch x 7-inch file box in my office that I use every once in a while. In it, there are various colored file cards with addresses, phone numbers and other such data.

The cards themselves are marked with colored dots and numerals in different corners, and the box has dividers in it that are alphabetical, numerical, and color-coded so they can be used to sort the cards in numerous ways. This little box lets me create a variety of tasks for patients, depending on their needs. For example, I can shuffle the cards, and the patient can file them according to the last names, alphabetically. Or the patient can divide all the individuals from the business enterprises. One can also file by zip code or by some identified characteristic on the card, such as nurse, tailor or coin collector.

Or one can choose all the red dots, blue dots or yellow dots, or those that appear on the right or left. This task requires fine-motor dexterity as well as perceptual acuity and cognitive ability that can be graded to meet the needs of the client. The task also can be expanded by using larger materials such as manila and accordion folders that require different physical skills to manipulate.

It is easy to see how this task can be extended to serve as a work-related test or training tool. One might also use such cards as the basis for typing a data set from which labels can be produced.

Sorting out a shoebox filled with extraneous office supplies is a great task for some people. When my granddaughter comes to the office, she delights in taking everything out of my desk drawers and sorting them out. The paper clips are sized and placed into different containers; the rubber bands are sorted and aligned, and the pens and pencils are separated. Markers are divided into 'permanent' and 'erasable'.

Pads of paper are placed in size order ranging from large ruled pads to sticky notes, which I find very helpful until I mess them up again.

Using a hole punch requires completely different skills and works different muscles depending upon whether one is standing or sitting. I can remember preparing for New Year's Eve by punching holes in paper to make confetti that I threw out the window of a six-story apartment house in Brooklyn at the stroke of midnight.

The most mundane tasks can be great fun when they have meaning. But they also may be applied to work. Today I use ring binders to keep all my course materials organized. Consequently, I am often forced to punch holes in stacks of paper and then file the papers according to the dates on which they will be needed. This task is easily converted to a purposeful and even meaningful therapy task.

Folding letters is a much-needed office task that requires a degree of precision if the product being prepared is to be fitted into an envelope. It is a repetitive task, with little cognitive demand, and can be incorporated into an assembly-line operation.

Pulling the address labels off a sheet, placing them onto envelopes, filling the envelopes and sorting by zip code can fill a number of hours, and provide satisfying work for some individuals, depending on their cognitive ability of their investment in the project. (If one were donating one's time to a charity or a political campaign through doing this task, the meaningfulness of the activity emerges.)

Reorganizing bookshelves is an important task and provides completely different demands. Standing before a high bookcase requires one to balance, reach, lift and bend, and also to make some decisions. I file my books by author, within certain large categories. But when they are borrowed and returned, people never put them back in the right places. Therefore, this job is forever available in my office; and its value is evident to someone who would volunteer for this work – if only they would.

Setting up and managing our petty cash account is a real task that could be easily simulated using receipts, a ledger, and a coin box. Calculation abilities are vital, as is the ability to keep track of items. This kind of activity, or even managing a checkbook, is one that most people find valuable, and with the software now available for businesses, this kind of task could be used to practice skills that apply to home or office.

Water sport in retirement

Originally published in *Advance for Occupational Therapy* May 20, 2002

Years ago I leaned to canoe, and I loved it. But I have not boated on the water under my own steam since that long ago time when I was a teenaged camper in New York State. This year the AOTA conference brought me to Florida, a paradise for water sports. Friends of mine invited us to kayak with them, and so we did among the mangrove trees on the Banana River.

Not only is Florida a site for water lovers, it is a place for retirees. My two friends Marc and Sue moved from Connecticut to Florida last August, where they are developing a new lifestyle. Prior to their retirement, Sue was a special education teacher; Marc was a business manager. They had raised three children who now had families of their own. Marc and Sue were used to active, demanding lives, with leisure usually limited to the weekends and vacations. Now they have days to fill. We spent only a few days with them, but I was fascinated by the many activities we shared with them and the other activities that they told us about.

They have a sailboat they pulled behind them on a trailer when they moved, intending to spend their days on the water. While they are experienced at boating, they are enrolling in classes to hone their skills and are checking out all the boating venues to find out the ones that are best. We received a tour of all the marinas and learned their pros and cons. And they brought us up to date on the whys and wherefores of surfboards, boogie boards, sail boards and kite boards.

When they are not moving along in the water, Marc and Sue find walks along the beach very gratifying and healthy, especially when the shells have come in. Their beautiful collection of shells is growing, and they know the names of all the shellfish, animals, birds – and even the butterflies – in their neighborhood. Remarkably, they have moved to a neighborhood filled with peacocks and peahens whose mating calls fill the night air. They are now waiting for the birds to molt so they can collect the feathers and begin a craft project with them.

Sue is a member of Mensa, and they attend many activities with this group. They play cards in the local bookstore on alternate Wednesday evenings, and meet with another group on Tuesdays of the other weeks.

Sue is also joining a club that is concerned with environmental issues. They will be taking water samples from estuary sites, and she will be learning to test the water scientifically. She is also planning to investigate a group that plants mangrove trees along the shoreline, restoring the original environment that was destroyed by less than careful development. Marc would rather fish.

Sue has become an assistant Girl Scout leader, resuming an interest she had when her children were younger, while Marc helps shuck the corn for their cookouts, since he loves to cook. And there's their granddaughter's soccer matches to check out. There are always guests to entertain. Family and friends are eager to visit their shorefront condominium.

Even these two retirees do talk about possibly returning to work some time down the road, however.

Not everyone is as gifted as Marc and Sue in finding meaningful activities. For some, retirement brings loneliness and depression. Many people need help in getting through the transition period. A work life has its schedule of events built in. Building a new 'time construction' takes a great deal of planning and courage. For some, it may take a 'tour guide'. What a suitable job for an occupational therapist, especially one who happens to live in a community with many retirees.

Occupational therapists have a long history of working with activity programming in nursing homes, using skills in interviewing people with limited abilities to identify old and new interests and weave them into a program to build a healthy leisure life. These same skills are needed to help healthy people build one. As occupational therapy moves into the community seeking non-traditional roles, retirement counseling is an area that deserves consideration.

We have the skills. The clients are out there. Give it a try. It might even be a good retirement job.

Did you ever want to be a '90s Johnny Appleseed?

Originally published in *Advance for Occupational Therapy* Sep. 15, 1997

Fall is coming. I can tell because the evenings are starting to be chilly, the leaves are beginning to blow about and there's a special smell in the air.

I can't wait until the apple trees are ripe with fruit. There's nothing like those crisp fall days when you finally find the time to take that walk in the fields to the orchard where the apples are shining red and ripe on the trees, as if they had been waiting for you all the time.

Bring a big basket with you, and a broom to knock down the fruit. Wear a hat to protect your head, as you spread a sheet on the ground while you reach as high as you can to swing away and watch the apples land and bounce.

Yes, some of them may bruise, but it sure is fun to see them come down. And don't forget the benefits of the exercise. Reach and bend, and reach and bend again. Pick them up. And reach and bend some more. Pile the fruit high into the basket. And when the basket is full, carry the apples back to the yard. And back to the orchard to get some more.

Best to bring a friend who will hold the other side of the basket as it swings between you. Friendships that are made like this last lifetimes.

Now over to the table where the fruit can be sorted. There is some to eat and some to cook. And what delicious things to cook.

Pies and applesauce are my favorites. They not only taste delicious, they make the kitchen smell so great.

Peel and slice until the bowl is full. Fill the pie pan with dough and then pile it high with fruit. Spread the sugar and the cinnamon on the top. Dot the fruit with butter. Now put a second crust of pie dough on top of the fruit. Pinch the edges of the dough together, score the crust with lovely designs. Pierce the crust with a fork. The sweet-smelling steam will fill the air as the pie bakes.

Now it's time to fill the pot to the brim with fruit that has been washed and trimmed. Whole apples work as well as cut ones, so decide for yourself.

Purists peel their fruit, but I keep the skins on; they make the sauce so pretty and pink. Set the pot to boil, lower the heat and kick back and enjoy the smell.

When the fruit is soft, use the ricer to strain the skins and seeds, separating them from the sauce. Add cinnamon or Jello, or keep it plain. Any way you do it, it tastes great.

Applesauce is always delicious no matter the recipe, and most delicious when you have gotten your hands into the job.

Pack the applesauce into sterile containers. Serve it warm if you are as impatient as I am.

Or wait for it to cool and watch everyone enjoy it. Serving your treasures to others is the most fun, especially when you see them lick their lips in pleasure.

If picking and cooking fruit is so much fun, why not share the experience with your patients? The outdoors is an excellent therapeutic environment, and connecting the outdoors to the indoors helps make the activities make sense.

Taking patients on an outing that results in such meaningful activity can be valuable in numerous ways. Meaningful activity, it seems to me, is activity that has lots of connected parts, where one can see the various parts of the task and how they relate to one another, thus giving meaning to the activity.

Such collaborative tasks make great group activities. By engaging in the unilateral and bilateral tasks of food preparation events (activities of daily living and homemaking training), patients also learn cause and effect, practice sequencing; take responsibility and share.

They can increase their strength and endurance while their hand skills grow. Their standing tolerance can improve – or their sitting balance, if that is what's needed. They can learn easy recipes that meet their dietary needs and give them pleasure preparing and eating.

And patients can learn skills that will be valued by people who are important to them. Which mom or dad won't be thought of as special if they show their families what wonders they can produce in the kitchen? For youngsters who need to learn skills they will use to live on their own, this is a great way to start building confidence and competence.

Why don't you start right now planning for the future? With your patients, plant a small apple tree in your center's front yard. It may take some time until it bears fruit. Maybe it won't be you who harvests that fruit. Maybe some other therapist and patients will benefit some years down the road. But if you never plant a tree, no one will ever enjoy the fruit. That's what Johnny Appleseed thought, and you know what an impact he had.

Pets and People

From before the time of recorded history, people have relied on animals for sustenance and comfort. This relationship between people and animals remains strong among people and their pets.

I, for one, live on a small farm in western New Jersey, a state just west of New York City, that is better known for its industrial and technological industries than its farms, although it is called the Garden State. In the thirty years we have lived on the farm, we have had a succession of animals sharing our home and property. We have housed many dogs and cats, and hosted lots of other creatures too. Over time, we have raised sheep, cattle, goats, horses and a variety of birds, including chickens and roosters of various breeds, as well as geese, guinea hens and peacocks.

Caring for these animals has given us great pleasure, yet it has been demanding at times. Shearing sheep is a tiresome job. Lambing Hampshires, the breed we raised, requires a willingness to withstand the harshest weather, as they give birth in the coldest months of the year, but watching the lambs romp in the spring makes it all worthwhile.

Aside from the pleasure they provide to us, the most important thing that our animals have brought to us was the responsibility they required. Learning to care for pets is a wonderful reality check for teaching children about the responsibility and caring that is also needed to raise human babies. Caring for the young of any breed of animals requires due diligence. Raising our children in an environment in which they assumed responsibility for the care of their animals made it clear to them and to us that animals impose their own structure on their caretakers. One must always be there to feed and water the animals, as they are totally dependent on you. In time, habits of responsibility become ingrained.

Recognizing that, it was a short step to notice that animals can be therapeutic in a variety of ways. A favorite dog sharing a bed with a sick child is comforting. Sometimes the companionship of a pet provides feelings of closeness and communication that are needed at times of sadness and stress. The same can be true for children and adults who are undergoing the stresses of illness and disability.

Following are two articles that focus on the therapeutic use of pets. These are merely examples of ways pets can be incorporated into a therapy program. I am sure you can think of other ways to expand your own use of animals as therapy tools.

Try some activities with man's best friend

Originally published in *Advance for Occupational Therapy* date unknown

At this year's Belgian Sheepdog National Specialty in Moodus, Connecticut, I thought about the many active opportunities that dogs and dog shows can provide for people with disabilities – both mental and physical – to attain accomplishment and a sense of great satisfaction.

Dog shows come in several varieties. There are conformation or beauty shows, and obedience or other performance events that emphasize agility or herding or field trials. Showing dogs is a fun activity in which everyone can find a niche. For example, grooming is a common activity for a dog and owner. Some dogs need to be brushed daily. Brushing a dog requires one to be able to grasp a brush and go to town, but even people with grasp dysfunction can do this if their brushes are adaptive with universal cuffs. Holding a brush and doing the extensive kind of brushing required by some breeds is bound to build muscles in the back, upper arm and shoulder. Brushing can be done sitting or standing, and both dog and human usually enjoy the activity. Some dogs do not require much brushing, except when they are shedding, which tends to happen for several weeks one or two times a year. Others, like afghan hounds, can take up to four hours to prepare for showing. Some breeds can look and feel great with a half-hour of brushing each evening, with owner and dog curled up together on the couch watching the evening news.

Most active show folk like to go to handling classes once a week. It's a wonderful way to make strong and lasting friendships. 'Dog people' are very apt to help one another get around unique problems, or help with transportation problems. People with disabilities will find that these people are supportive and capable of understanding special needs. After all, each of the dogs has special needs as well. Some are quick to learn, some slow; some are skilled, some are not. The same is true with people, and dog folk recognize that.

The meaningful relationship built up between dogs and their handlers has great value for therapy. People who have difficulty in relating to other people can learn to build positive relationships with dogs. It is important to recognize that dogs are dependent on their owners for love as well as sustenance.

Some youngsters with behavioral problems respond very well to the lasting feelings that develop when they are totally responsible for a dog that cares about them without compromise. Troubled youngsters who have difficulty communicating verbally can begin to learn to communicate with their dogs, extending this skill more broadly over time to people. Learning to be responsible for an animal leads to learning to be responsible in many other areas of living.

It's gratifying to watch an individual with physical disabilities in a wheelchair engage in obedience competition with his or her dog. The competition scoring is based on the performance of dog and handler as a working team. Points are deducted exactly the same for all participants in the competition, regardless of their use of adaptive aids. Dogs must heel on and off lead, come when called, stand and be examined and sit or lie without breaking away. And the sense of accomplishment is the same for able-bodied or disabled. Along with the exercise, it is hard to remain depressed when your favorite pal takes the time to amuse you.

One of our retired champions was adopted by a nursing home and spent several years in residence there, providing great comfort and pleasure. A friend of mine who works at a residence for people with mental retardation hosts a dog show at her site each year. Those of the residents who are capable have the opportunities to show a dog and compete in a match competition operated much like the Special Olympics. Dogs, handlers, families and staff all have a great time.

Only your imagination probably limits the number of therapeutic opportunities that dogs and dog showing provides. Try it. You'll like it!

Are pets the therapy tool your practice is missing?

Originally published in *Advance for Occupational Therapy* Feb. 19, 1996

Animals are a regular part of many people's lives. In fact, animal lovers structure much of their lives around their pets, creating many activities on their behalf: long walks, periods of brushing, visits to places where their animals can socialize, etc. And for those who love animals, being separated from them because of illness or disability is a great hardship. For these reasons, animals are wonderful additions to the therapy toolbox.

They respond affectionately to those who take care of them.

Touching pets and communicating with them has been found to lower blood pressure and increase longevity. And because they need attention, animals instill responsibility and a feeling of being needed.

A number of years ago, my colleague Pat Stollmack, MA, OTR, discussed with me her intention to obtain a dog for the New Jersey county psychiatric hospital where she worked. I raise and show Belgian sheepdogs and offered her a puppy from the next litter knowing there could be no better role for one of our pups. Belgian sheepdogs like people, are hardy and easy to care for. (I registered the puppy as Breines Onyx Treasure, hoping they would call her 'OT'.)

Pat took the pup to the hospital each day and brought her home every night so she would feel attached to a family. Ignoring my devious plan for the name, however, Pat engaged everyone in selecting a name for the puppy. She walked the dog from ward to ward, and put up signs with the puppy's picture on them, announcing that there would be a vote to select the name. Everyone had the opportunity to suggest one. Committees met to organize these suggestions.

For some residents, this was the first time they had expressed any interest in their environment, and for others, it was their first decision-making event. In due course the vote was held and the puppy was forevermore dubbed Midnight. She made her home at the hospital for many years and was a meaningful addition to the program.

Another of our dogs took up residence in a nursing home. She had been shown widely in breed and obedience, and was used to being with strangers. We set up a trial period. We began by making visits to the home, introducing Yummy to everyone. Once she was familiar with the home she stayed for longer and longer periods on her own. Finally, it was time to move in.

The maintenance man built a small picket fence in a corner of the recreation room so Yummy could rest and have privacy when she wanted it. Everyone agreed that when Yummy was resting, she was not to be disturbed.

Staff and residents volunteered to be responsible for various aspects of her care, feeding, exercise and grooming, etc. Yummy and those residents thrived on each other's company. The dog went on rounds with the nurses. She knew who wanted her visits and who did not. She waited for the elevator and got on and off at will. Yummy had certain favorites and made visiting them a part of her own daily rounds.

If you are interested in using dogs in your clinic, one good resource is Therapy Dogs International. Dog owners in this organization train their dogs to visit nursing homes and other sites. The owners can usually be reached by contacting your local kennel club.

Birds, hamsters, guinea pigs and cats also make good 'therapists'. Remember, live animals must be taken care of every day, even on weekends; it's a good idea to involve everyone in the decision-making process at the outset, so their cooperation is assured when you need their help. But the buck stops with you. If you feel the responsibility might be too much, decide that before you adopt an animal. If you do decide to adopt one after careful consideration, you will enjoy having a tool at hand that expands your professional repertoire immeasurably.

Occupational Technology and Occupational Therapy

Occupational therapy is sometimes hard to explain because it is so comprehensive and extensive, particularly in terms of the tools we use in therapy. One interesting way to view the profession is to examine it in parallel with the activities human beings have invented and adapted from the beginning of pre-history through to the modern era.

Just as human history reveals the acquisition of skills in ever-advancing technologies, from those of earliest humans (e.g. clay, leather, basketry), through those of the industrial era (e.g. carpentry, metalcrafts, printing), to those of the modern era (e.g. computers, electronics, videography), the tools of occupational therapy practice extend from 'clay to computers' and beyond.

Occupational therapy began as a formalized profession during the industrial revolution. It was a time in which society incorporated industrial tasks and products into a new and changing world.

At the same time, some aspects of society recognized the hazards of industrialization. These concerns were reflected by the ideas and practices of the Arts & Crafts movement, which coincidently had a role in the development of the profession. The profession adopted many of the handcrafts which stemmed from an earlier period but which were familiar during the industrial era, adapting them for various therapeutic purposes.

All activities invented to that point in time became accepted professional tools. We adopted the activity analysis of industrialization and applied this notion to the arts and crafts, despite the fact that their underlying principles emerged from different sources and reflected divergent beliefs.

Since that time, society has undergone a technological revolution that has introduced many new instruments and gadgets that affect health, both negatively and positively. Today, the daily lives of many people utilize many technological items. The industrialized world has become a world of computers and electronics applied to life's activities. Banks, supermarkets and various methods of transportation have become part of everyday life. People communicate and shop on the Internet, and use automatic cash machines. They shop in markets that use computers to calculate bills and monitor merchandise. Grandparents see their new grandbabies moments after birth, through the magic of digital photography. Telephones and television are part of almost everyone's lives, and even these change rapidly, encouraging people to keep up with the newest items. The mobile cell phone is now a worldwide phenomenon, even in countries where poverty is great.

If the tools of everyday living are the tools used by our patients, they are necessarily the tools of occupational therapists. This is understandable, since we help patients to gain skills in the tasks they need to perform in their daily lives. Therapists have shown no hesitation in making these tools their own. Many of these new activities have been brought into the occupational therapy compendium.

Following are several articles that describe some technological applications used in modern life and in occupational therapy practice, reflecting how technology keeps changing and influencing practice. Every day brings new inventions and new applications for therapy. I have come to call our knowledge and use of the tools for therapy 'Occupational Technology', recognizing that they include all those technological features of activity that range 'from clay to computers' and then some.

A chapter of this sort is out of date even before it is written, given the state of modern technology. Changes in tools occur daily, and no one can anticipate which new inventions will next become part of daily living. One would hope that these ideas will be viewed as metaphorical, not explicit in terms of current practice, since we live in a constantly changing world that alters rapidly each day.

But who is better equipped to deal with change and convert these ideas to new and creative notions than a practitioner who is guided by the principles of adaptation?

Occupational technology, past, present and future

Estelle B. Breines, Tamara Avi-Itzhak, Meryl M. Picard and Elizabeth Torcivia
Previously published in http://gradmeded.shu.edu/occtech

Throughout history, advances in technology have changed the occupational experiences, roles and skills of human beings. This has been true since humans first walked the earth, and continues to be so. And with each new invention the process of adaptation is replicated, bringing us to an era marked by rapid technological change (Breines, 1995).

The technological growth available at the beginning of this new millennium is comparable to the industrial revolution that heralded the transition from the 19th to the 20th centuries. Sweeping changes in how we perform daily tasks are commonplace. These changes are anticipated to continue as advances in technology escalate. The occupations in which humans engage as time passes will change beyond our current imaginations (Post, 1996) and will outstrip the remarkable adaptations that have structured our past. And with these developments, human lives will change. These changes are important for occupational therapists to understand if we are to facilitate positive change in clients as they adapt to the new worlds in which they find themselves. To affect this understanding, a comprehensive analysis of the effects of technology on occupation needs to be undertaken.

An historical perspective

From the beginning of human history, technological advances in the use of the environment contributed to the health and well-being of individuals and societies. Natural materials, varying from place to place in the world according to the particulars of climate and terrain, were creatively adapted to support lives in many different ways. As an example, palm fronds from the tropics and pine needles from the mountains were constructed into baskets, each of which served similar occupational purposes within their respective cultures.

Skill in the use of various techniques and materials were developed within each environment, and were incorporated into the lives of the community, time permitting their testing. The time required to accept or reject these new notions was extensive. Adapting new phenomena into the occupational repertoire was controlled by their acceptance by the community. Taboos were not easily broken.

As skills were acquired, those that benefited the community were retained. Unsuccessful ideas were weeded out as they were proven dysfunctional, while healthful ideas thrived. For example, the technology associated with the removal of poison from manioc (a poisonous but otherwise nutritive vegetable grown in the tropics) (American Museum of Natural History, 2002) was undoubtedly developed over an extended period of trial and error so that the nutritional benefits it provides are not diminished by its risk to health. Time allowed this refinement to occur.

As new skills were acquired, they came to provide sustenance and meaning to persons living in that society. Earliest peoples, as they grew to understand how to make pots, baskets, ropes and nets, clothing, weapons and other artifacts, developed these through sophisticated constructional technologies (Breines, 1995). For example, firing clay and curing leather are complex technological skills. Expertise in their manufacture requires a knowledge of materials and techniques that takes many years to acquire.

Members of the community learned their roles in the performance of each occupation, and performed those roles effectively, parent teaching child, into the next generations, thus assuring their mutual survival and well-being through an oral tradition. In time, driven by their quest for certainty (Dewey, 1929) and the irrepressible creativity with which humans are endowed, technologies of agriculture, metals and mechanization were developed. Each new advance led to still further adaptive invention, brought forth by the creativity of humankind. Methods advanced along with materials, and with each new formulation societies and cultures changed, each change serving as a harbinger for future change.

Evolving technological influences

From multiple generations affording refinement of new inventions, to an individual lifetime in which a new invention was ideated, expressed and integrated, we have come to a time of such rapid change that children's skills often exceed those of the parents. It is not uncommon for today's parents to look for offspring to program the VCR or load the newest software. We are now facing a world in which occupational adaptation (Schkade and Schultz, 1992; Schultz and Schkade, 1992) is evolving beyond the imagination of any one person or community. Occupational forms (Nelson, 1988) are altering. Who could have believed a few short years ago that seven young boys of varying ages could spend hours together in play, each engaged with their own Game Boy, interacting only to share disks? What impact will this have on their physical and mental capacity and their occupational roles as providers later in life? What impact on society will come from children refining their skills beyond that of their parents? Only time will tell.

One of the major effects of this rapid escalation of technology is the expansion of communication, which itself contributes to further technological change. No longer is our ability to communicate inventiveness restricted by geography. When people were isolated from one another by mountains, rivers, oceans and ice, their creations remained unique and apart. Cultures and languages developed along with artifacts, bounded by geographical limitations. It was only when people breached the hazards of travel that these unique ideas were spread. Communication was hard won.

Today, daily communication with all parts of the earth and beyond is available to the average person in the modern world, and in many parts of the third world as well. Radio, television, e-mail, the Internet, LAN connection, cellular phones, teleconferencing and beepers are within reach of many people. With new advances in miniaturization, portability and digitalization these items are readily available at all times, encouraged in the expansion of their use by diminishing costs to the consumer. Increasingly, these technologies are linked to each other (New York Times, 2000b), adding to a wide array of available products. With such ease of communication, each idea becomes part of the collective conscious (Jung, 1964), changing the world rapidly as we inform one another of each new technological advance. The integration of the newest technologies with ancient and varying cultures is a phenomenon that is replicating throughout the world (Swerdlow, 1999).

The Internet, once restricted to government research and educational institutions, now provides synchronous or asynchronous communication, launching chat rooms, e-groups and educational opportunities, and a vast array of relevant and often irrelevant information. Internet and cellular etiquette are argued about and new customs are adopted as social networks dictate. Schools and classrooms are equipped with computers, facilitating communication among students throughout the world, even those who previously could not communicate at all because of physical incapacity. Distance learning and other technological advances are now features of education. Work now encompasses telecommuting with increased use of home-based offices. The incorporation of these ideas into governmental regulation is being established. Secretary of Labor Alexis Herman has called for a national dialogue to discuss employee safety in this new century, including telecommuting issues (US Department of Labor, January 5, 2000).

Economic changes have also been associated with technological advance. In 1999 one saw the NASDAQ, the home of technology stock, rise to become the darling of Wall Street and then fall precipitously in 2000. Individuals now can easily govern their own investments from home, sometimes referred to as a new 'cottage industry' (Shanzel, 2000). The country as a whole has moved to a service economy affecting worker roles. Therapists have seen billing and scheduling become computerized. The MDS-2 must be electronically 'locked in' and transferred to the states by deadlines to insure Medicare compliance. Outcome software, statistical packages and productivity management increasingly are technology-based. But we are uncertain of the long range effects of this vast technology on occupational roles and health within society and culture.

Effects on health

As the newest technologies bring creative opportunities for living lives meaningfully and fully, new problems are being created which demand inventive solutions. The world is shrinking, but the adaptive problems people are experiencing are expanding. This expansion puts health at risk in ways we are only beginning to understand and cannot really anticipate. Uncertainty about the future has imbedded fear into the general public. Brain tumors associated with portable phones are among the newest unproven projections of ill health. Fear of the health effects of communication towers is as of great concern as the notion of fear of the unknown itself, as the new technologies rapidly emerge. Air travel speeds viruses around the world, bringing disease to and from the farthest reaches of the world (Johnson, 1996; Shilts, 1987). Hours spent seated in virtual immobilization exposed to implements that reputedly exude radiation have yet unknown effects on health. We understand that space travel in gravity-free environments results in diminished strength and impaired balance. We do not know its further effects.

Cumulative trauma injuries, while evident well into ancient times (Molleson, 1994), are now caused by new tools, effected largely by the speed with which these tools are used. We are pushing the envelope of our thus evolved physical capacity to perform. Understanding human endeavor to prevent these disorders requires an in-depth knowledge of the interaction among physical and mental capacities and intentions, with the tangible and social environment, and the recognition of this interaction as a developmental and evolutional phenomenon (Breines, 1981, 1986a, 1995). The field of ergonomics has begun to address some of these issues, but ergonomics and assistive technology is not the entire story.

Effects on labor and society

In the same way that technology has impacted on health, it is also impacting on the workforce. 'By 2006, nearly half of all US workers will be employed in industries that produce or intensively use information technology, products and services' (US Department of Commerce, 1999, p. 1A).

The gap in skills and education between entry level and executive management positions has widened resulting in increasingly unequal earnings (US Department of Labor, 1999). Not all Americans have equal access to technology (Rockefeller University, 1999), further widening the gap between different levels of society.

Jobs that were primarily hand operated now demand the integration of technological skill. The mechanic now utilizes diagnostic and hand held computers to adjust computerized systems in automobiles. Federal Express drivers use portable hand held computers to track delivery of packages from point of origin to point of destination. The local supermarket computes inventory, discounts and customer buying patterns from a computer database.

A recent review of the classified advertisements regarding computer technology in the *New York Times* (2000b) reveals that jobs for temporary workers and administrative assistants now require expertise in Word, Excel and Power Point. Jobs are listed for programmers, web programmers, LAN administrators, hardware technicians, software sales engineers and Information Technology directors. Virtually none of these occupations were identified ten years ago, while traditional jobs are being done in new ways. Recognizing this remarkable change in society and the labor force is particularly critical for occupational therapy, as it is our purpose to return people to former and new occupational roles.

Occupational therapy and occupational technology

Clearly, the breadth of human inventiveness is expanding exponentially through myriad technological advances. The advent of modern technology has changed occupation immeasurably and with its continued evolution, further changes are anticipated. There is every indication that we are on the cusp of inventive technologies that will affect the occupational lives of everyone in the modern world to at least as great an extent as has already been experienced. It is less than a generation since computers became available to the public, and the changes we have experienced in that short time are enormous. Atkinson and Court (1998) report, 'It has taken only seven years for the Internet to be adopted by 30% of Americans, compared to 17 years for television and 38 years for the telephone' (p. 19). There is every anticipation that comparable changes will continue.

The implications of these changes for occupational therapy are stunning. Each day brings with it new ways of living, and with it new and potential dangers. It behooves us to prepare for this understanding (Post, 1996) by investigating the effects of this phenomenon on health and wellness.

Occupational therapists have had a long history of understanding and developing competence in technologies and the implications of these technologies for occupational performance and health. The tools and media which instruct us in adaptive capacity have served as a foundation for understanding of human occupation. From the beginning of our profession to the modern era, occupational therapists have trained in the competence required to analyze and manipulate media through occupations of every description (Breines, 1995, 2002), recognizing that this skill enables us to provide our patients with adaptive solutions to their unique occupational dysfunctions.

Hammel and Luebben (1996) applied Uniform Terminology to the analysis of assistive technology. Our literature discusses low tech and high tech solutions (Anson, 1997; Bain and Leger, 1997; Jacobs and Bettencourt, 1995; Mann and Lane, 1995; Struck, 1995), and our expertise instructs us in the appropriate use of each, alone and in combination. Technology is a tool for occupation, and is a tool for occupational therapy (Smith et al., 1992).

With each new technological advance, its application to occupation and occupational dysfunction throughout the life span made its way into our professional repertoire. Our curricula incorporated knowledge of technology from the outset (Post, 1996). We have not stood still. Each new development civilization has offered has been incorporated into the therapeutic repertoire of the occupational therapy practitioner.

This is an appropriate venture for the profession, as the occupations of patients are necessarily those of therapists themselves. The ability of patients to perform their life tasks is largely dependent upon therapists' ability to facilitate performance. In preparation for this responsibility, occupational therapists in their education process learn to perform and analyze occupations of every description as a foundation for understanding their adaptive potential. These occupations span the breadth of technological advances that humans developed over the course of history. Computers and modern technology components are as important a tool for therapy as the traditional media introduced at the outset of the profession (Breines, 1995).

A call for action

Understanding the relationship between traditional and modern technologies serves as a foundation for understanding occupational technology because it structures an understanding of future change. We are entering an era of change that demands attention if we are to understand the needs of our clients. Adopting occupational technology as a recognized and inherent part of occupational therapy's education and research will contribute to the profession's enhancement of work, play and self care, in wellness, dysfunction and adaptive living. Beginning a formalized study of the influences of occupational technology on human occupation and health will strengthen and validate the profession's expertise in this phenomenon.

The new art of videography

Originally published in *Advance for Occupational Therapy* May 15, 1995

In a psychiatric unit in Wyckoff, New Jersey, Diana Hunt, OTR, is using the modern art of videography in the most creative ways to bring youngsters together in meaningful activity.

One of her groups made a series of instructional 'how-to' tapes. Another wrote a screenplay that group members costumed, dramatized and taped. Still another group used the videocamera to record events in the community, then brought the tape back to be played for those residents who did not have the opportunity to attend the events. In addition, Hunt's teens have recorded themselves in simulated job interviews.

Because video viewing is so much a part of their society, youngsters today find it very meaningful. And with the advent of new hand-held cameras, and the easy availability of the VCR, videotaping has opened up new vistas for therapeutic practices. Drama has been a useful clinical tool for some time now; having the opportunity to act out behaviors and then to examine them on videotape greatly extends that usefulness, for this is a medium that lends itself to self-review as well as feedback from others.

But videography is also a good home-education tool for the rehabilitation center, the geriatric center or the pediatric environment. How many times have you wished you could go home with patients to make sure they could do the special techniques you spent so long teaching them? Well, just tape the instructions and send them along, or tape the patients doing the activities properly, so they will have a visual reminder. And not only will the patient be reminded, but the family and others as well.

And how about that documentation you are always needing to provide? Nothing beats a videotape of 'before' and 'after' to show that the patient is benefiting from occupational therapy services. Nor are team meetings such deadly dull events if you can show your colleagues how and why you use the tools you do.

Good videography, like any art, requires education and practice. There are many different kinds of cameras, and an equal number of devices to play the tapes on – the commonly used 1/2-inch VHS, the older Betamax, and the newer 8 mm. format. If you are planning to purchase a videocamera and/or a VCR, be certain the various pieces of equipment you get are compatible with one another. You may have to make choices based on price, system, size and weight, or available features such as in-camera labeling devices.

If a number of different people have access to the equipment, they will also want to learn to use it well. It is a good idea to copy the instructions and file them in an equipment library in the department.

Put a check list in with the camera listing all the parts, so everyone can be sure to put the equipment away in its entirety. (For example, it is often necessary to use specific cables to transmit from the camera to the VCR. Without those cables, you will not be able to proceed, so determine a way of keeping track of all parts.)

Practice operating the camera before you plan to use it for some critical purpose. As with all activities, it is necessary for the user to build confidence in all the procedures to be effective. You might want to begin to learn how to use it at a clinic party.

I'm sure you can think of many more ways to use the video camera as a professional tool than I have suggested here. Good luck and have fun.

Chasing the perfect button

Originally published in *Advance for Occupational Therapy* March 25, 2002

My interests in occupational technology have driven me to peruse some new documents on a regular basis lately. For one, I make sure to read the Circuits section of the *New York Times*, which appears every Thursday. Circuits is devoted to introducing new ideas in technology.

Making sure to read the paper every Thursday is not an easy feat for me. I car pool, and since I drive every other day, I only get to read the paper on alternate days. But I am sure to catch Circuits, no matter what. There's always a new goodie described there, but I turn the page and forget it knowing full well that my pocket can never keep up with the newest technological advances. I remain delighted with my Dell desktop computer at home and my IBM laptop at school. I'd better get used to them – no one is gong to replace them too soon. But I still like to check out the new stuff.

In reading the *Times* last week (sometimes my reading backs up), I came to realize that not everything in Circuits is new. What is new is the way we approach things. In a delightful article by Michelle Slatalla entitled, 'In Tender Pursuit of the Perfect Button' (Feb. 21, 2002: G4), I learned a new way to shop for old stuff. As a committed crafts person, I've always taken great pleasure in discovering the many little treasures one could find on a walk through New York City's garment center, or a flea market almost anywhere in the world. Here I've found beads, yarn and other such stuff. And wherever I found them, I couldn't resist touching and feeling these treasures.

But this new way to shop – although probably not new to many of you – never occurred to me before with regard to craft materials, so committed have I been to shopping in the real world. Apparently there is a network out there of people like myself who are also entranced by 'objects d'art' which are not only beautiful in and of themselves, but are the components for many other treasures.

Slatalla tells a story about the relationship she builds with a friend named Nancy. The pair have developed 'an old-fashioned vaudeville routine'. Nancy gives her old stuff to Michelle because she sees it as useless, and Michelle dreams up ways to perk it up or use it differently. Nancy responds by making snide remarks about smelling mildew, or other such negative comments.

On one occasion, Michelle decides that she'll dress up a hand-me-down sweater by replacing the old buttons with exotic new buttons. The problem is that Michelle can't find them in her usual haunts, so she is forced to search the Web. In the article, she provides a list of Web sites, 'where you can buy an assortment of more than 600 buttons for $5.77' and other wonderful items:

- www.victorialouise.com
- www.laceforless.com
- www.jkmribbon.com
- www.buttons4u.com
- www.rhinestonz.co.nz

Now that my eyes are open, there's no stopping me from browsing the Web to find craft items. Now I can find more stuff than I'll ever have room for. The only drawback is that I can't touch them before I buy them and that takes away much of the fun. So I may be protected to some extent.

Once Michelle gets her Internet buttons, she indulges her 'can you top this?' attitude. She invites Nancy to dinner just so she can show off her brand new renovated sweater.

Do I need to make the connection to occupational therapy here? I think not. But just in case I am wrong, how about these ideas: communication and sharing, motivation, fine motor skills, mobility, pride and satisfaction, self care, economics, and so on. You pick the one that works for you.

CSU's creative links to human health

Originally published in *Advance for Occupational Therapy* Nov. 28, 1998

I had a computer printout on my desk for more than a month – a note from the Internet that had the address of a website that sounded interesting. In fact, it sounded like fun. But pressures of time had kept me from responding to the e-mail because I had so many 'more important' things to do. At least I thought they were more important.

Finally, fed up with the explosion of paper on my desk, I determined to go through all the pages that had piled up one by one and deal with them. And so, with my newfound systematic approach to order, I came upon the note with the Web address on it. I booted up the computer and punched in the address: http://www.scu.edu.au/faculty/health/cmhealth/creative.

I had to wait a few minutes for the site to emerge, because its origins were on the other side of the world. The paper held this intriguing invitation: 'It is with pleasure that I invite everyone to view the web site created by Charles Sturt University (Albury, Australia) undergraduate occupational therapy students. The Web site shows and describes the work produced by the students for a creative links exhibition they produced last year. It also discusses some of the theory and work behind the scenes.' The letter was signed by Claire Wilding, lecturer in occupational therapy.

Opening this website was like finding a precious jewel. After all, much of what is on the Net is not worth much, and finding the good stuff usually requires a lot of sorting.

On these very special pages, I was able to view photographs of the many wonderful creations the students had produced, organized by topic of interest and accompanied by descriptive documentation of each project, offered by its student artist. Each presentation was accompanied by a photo of the artist.

The site is beautifully constructed. It grasps the essential elements of active occupation and translates them into an understanding of the importance of occupation for human expression. It also ties the essence of these concepts to the delivery of occupational therapy services. Here is an eloquent expression of what makes occupational therapy special. This site nobly uplifts occupation, in my mind.

Is it the naivete of young people that allows them to see so clearly what has become obscured for many older therapists? Is it that students who are given the time to explore can find answers that are not so readily available to busy professionals?

All I know is that I, also, am proud of my identity as an occupational therapist, proud even of our basketmaking.

If we as occupational therapists do not value such fundamental skills and the link they have to health, we will be sold down the river (in a basket). We cannot expect anyone else to respect us if we do not respect ourselves. That means we must be experts in how human beings act, act on their environments and act with others. In order to become experts we need to learn, once again, to do. And we need to teach others how to do. We will never be able to do this with proficiency unless we have pride in that doing.

The students at CSU clearly have learned this. Their teachers have taught it. And their patients will benefit from it. Bravo, CSU. You have reminded us all of something valuable. Keep it up. We have lots to learn.

I'm not gong to give you examples of what I found on this Web site. To find out, you'll have to explore it yourself. But I am adding the Web site to my required reading for next term. I suggest you add it to yours as well.

What could you do in the clinic with a 'peace' of paper?

Originally published in *Advance for Occupational Therapy* Sep. 18, 1995

Several weeks ago, knowing of my interest in crafts, Emily Weinstein, an occupational therapist, doctoral student and ADVANCE field correspondent, came to visit me with a videotape to review.

The tape, produced and directed by her friend Daniel L. Hess, was a demonstration tape for making origami (the old Japanese art of paper-folding). It was titled 'The Peace of Paper'.

The videotape was full of good techniques, clearly and charmingly demonstrated; it displayed the use of such everyday materials as index and business cards as well as traditional origami paper.

Folding instructions were delivered in conjunction with some delightful tales and games, making the tape fun to watch. It made me want to pull out some paper and begin to learn these new techniques.

I could clearly see how the techniques, and even the storytelling that went with them, could be used in therapy. It occurred to me when I saw the video that there are probably many therapists who would introduce crafts into the clinic if they only knew how to do the crafts.

Depending upon the school they attended, they may or may not have been educated to use crafts in therapy. Some schools encourage students to learn these activities on their own, and while some students undoubtedly do, many do not, leaving a hole in their education.

But it is never too late to learn new skills. Even therapists whose education included crafts can learn new and interesting techniques. Over the years I have seen many well-produced videotapes showing skills used in doing crafts. We now have available to us, through videography, the kind of expertise that can help the therapist become proficient in any number of craft techniques.

In fact, because of their wide availability, it is a good idea to begin to accumulate a library of instruction videos on crafts for the clinic.

One tape I have used in the classroom and lab demonstrates the techniques used in warping a loom. I purchased it at my local weaving shop, where I had the opportunity to review several tapes before purchasing this one. In class, the group viewed selected sections of the tape so they could see how weaving is done on a four-harness loom. Those students who wanted to experience how to warp the loom themselves were able to set up the videotape, using it as an individual tutor. By starting and stopping the tape as needed, they were able to learn at their own pace.

Therapists can use this method for all sorts of craft techniques. It requires an investment of personal time, but all kinds of education require that. If using these techniques is valuable to patients, then learning them is a worthwhile investment and a professional obligation on the part of the therapist. It is also fun to learn new activities, and occupational therapists who work so hard during their workdays can relax and enjoy such things on evenings and weekends.

The videotape can also be used to instruct patients. They should watch the tape from beginning to end, then start and stop it to review techniques as they work. Moreover, in the same way people use exercise tapes as motivators, patients can borrow tapes to use at home between therapy sessions, to encourage them to do therapy at home.

In addition to using commercially prepared films, it may be useful to tape therapists instructing patients, and patients performing the activities. Sometimes watching oneself work is a good reminder of the process being used.

You can even add to the videotape as a record of patient performance. What is sometimes difficult to document in writing is easily accomplished with a visual record. Having such a record also will provide data to be used as a basis for research, helping us to understand how activity is valuable in rehabilitation.

Teaching and Learning through Activity

Creating an occupational therapist requires a set of items, ideas and people. First and foremost is the student. Second is the teacher with his/her ideas, interests and experience. Third are the tools for learning, among which are the tangible items of the environment along with the patients from whom we learn. While these are listed here hierarchically, they are in actuality an integrated set, each contributing to the learning event.

Designing an academic learning experience demands that there be a clear recognition of the goals for learning. In addition, a defined sequence of experiences can make all the difference. In the case of the occupational therapist, the principle of learning through doing, proffered by John Dewey, the educational philosopher and pragmatist, is the leading principle for learning, for this is the principle which guides practice.

Occupational therapy is guided by the ideas of purposeful, active occupation. It is best to learn according to the same principles that guide one's professional interests. If we believe in these ideas, then we should acknowledge their application to the process of learning. After all, occupational therapy practice is as much an educational experience as it is a therapeutic event. Virtually all of practice requires the therapist to teach and the patient to learn. So the teaching/learning process has to be learned by the student therapist in order to gain proficiency as a practitioner.

Where to start and how best to formulate the educational experience are the questions. These articles look at the laboratory activities of the classroom, the clinical education experiences of a number of students and teachers and some of the problems some colleagues and I have encountered over time that tend to contribute to or interfere with the learning process. Needless to say, there is a heavy emphasis on active occupation (read that as crafts). I hope you will gather some ideas here for your own learning and teaching.

Students' appreciation of crafts is not universal

Originally published in *Advance for Occupational Therapy* June 12, 1995

Some people look at crafts as arts. Others look at crafts for the skills they offer. Occupational therapy educators see other things in crafts in the curriculum.

It has long been my contention that of all the academic experiences, the activities lab most closely parallels the clinical experience. For that reason, in the environment of the activities laboratory, it is most evident which students will be successful therapists and which skills students need to develop. Just as occupational therapy reveals how patients will perform in their lives, the laboratory reveals how future therapists will perform in their work roles. The laboratory can teach students many skills they will need as therapists beyond the apparent skills needed to perform the given activities.

My own class approaches activity from an historical/philosophical perspective, somewhat unique for a class on 'doing'. The class emphasizes that activities are meaningful for people in the context of their culture and environment. Learning activities within that context helps students to understand how activities developed to meet the needs of society, and how that meaningfulness may or may not be relevant to individuals in the modern world. Crafts and other activities are taught in the approximate sequence in which they were devised, from the Stone Age, Bronze Age, and Iron Age into the Industrial and Technological eras to emphasize the initial role of these activities as work, and for some, their continued use in industry to date. From this perspective, students learn about the world of work and their own role in preparing patients for that world.

Beyond recognizing that crafts were initially performed as work roles, and may now be art forms or employment, students learn that they vary markedly in their own appreciation of these activities. This unique appreciation for these activities is most significant.

Students are encouraged to express their dislikes as well as their likes, so their classmates will understand that their own perspectives are not universal. It is very common for people to assume that their own views hold true for others. By exposing them to differences in likes and dislikes, students are led to understand that one cannot predict who will like or dislike specific activities, and that the uniqueness of individuals must be respected. Furthermore, their responsibility as therapists is to meet patients' needs, so they have an obligation to learn a variety of activities that may not be their own particular preference, but may be useful in therapy because of interests expressed by patients.

Some therapists have suggested that specific activities have inherent qualities that are therapeutic, and that these qualities could form the basis for a prescriptive approach to activity. My own observations of students, who represent a normative population, reveal that students respond uniquely and unpredictably to different activities. I can't help but believe that their responses parallel those of patients. This would certainly be an interesting and informative topic for research.

Another phenomenon that students learn can be summarized as uncertainty/certainty. Each week or two, as each new activity is introduced, students characteristically are anxious, deliberate, cautious, and the class is palpably silent except for the sound of their work. As students proceed, they begin to perform automatically, and the humming begins. Groups form, chatter increases, and laughter emerges. They serve as teachers and critics, facilitators and friends. Uncertainty/certainty is introduced as a topic for discussion so students can come to understand an unfamiliar task, and how competence contributes to self confidence, affect and interaction behaviors. Learning unfamiliar or uncertain tasks is what occupational therapy patients are engaged in. Learning how it feels to encounter uncertainty helps the student to develop empathy, and learning how it feels to accomplish a task successfully shows the special qualities of tangible accomplishment that underlies occupational therapy.

Another aspect of learning is that of developing confidence with tools and media. With a sufficiently varied set of activities, one can learn how to manipulate just about every type of medium. Clay, leather, wood and computers are tangibly different. Learning how to manipulate each of them extrapolates into skill with other media of similar qualities. Developing skill in various media prepares students to use media for such things as therapeutic crafts or for adapting equipment or environments. Being skilled in manipulating a varied environment also can prepare them for unanticipated activities the future will bring.

One of the reasons occupational therapy is effective is that it relies on 'doing' as opposed to talking about doing.

Learning to do activity teaches about activity and its influences on people. Learning how students respond to activity is a basis for understanding how all people respond to activity, and can be extrapolated to how patients respond. The activity laboratory provides the environment for students to learn from themselves and from one another, so as to prepare them for their future roles as clinicians.

Will occupational therapists who use crafts please stand

Originally published in *Advance for Occupational Therapy* March 18, 1996

For many of us who teach, the best we can hope for is that the students have learned something from us that they can take with them. So when one hears from a former student, it is always a pleasure. And when one hears from that student that he or she has learned something found to be valuable, it is a great pleasure indeed.

The other day I received a letter from Calista Hendrikson, a former student of mine, asking if there was a special interest group for students and therapists interested in the use of crafts in therapy. What a novel idea, I thought, but I had to answer that I knew of no such group. However, there's no reason why we can't start one.

I fully expected that the suggestion would fall on deaf ears because it meant that a degree of extra work would be involved, and we are all so busy. Much to my surprise, the next letter I received included a list of several of Calista's classmates whom she thought also would be interested.

So now I reason that if a few are interested, perhaps many would be. On Calista's behalf I write this column as a request to those of you out there who think that such a group would be valuable to you. For now, I am happy to be the contact person for such a group through the Activity Notebook at OT ADVANCE or via my e-mail address: (breinees@shu.edu). If we find there is enough interest, I can put you in touch with one another and we'll take it from there. AOTA conference is coming up, and perhaps we can get together in Chicago.

Judging from the comments I get here and there, there are many occupational therapists who still use crafts as therapeutic tools and who think such activities are valuable. 'Coming out' as crafts proponents may help us all better examine why we are crafts users – at work or in our private lives. For if we can understand why we find crafts important to us, we will be reminded why they work in the clinic.

If there are numbers of us who advocate these tools, it may no longer be necessary to defend ourselves when we want to use them in practice. Creating a group would give us a body of human resources through whom dialogue and research are possible. Recent research into the use of creative activities in occupational therapy is in short supply. I do believe we have yet to examine why human beings find it important to solve tangible problems and obtain satisfaction through creative accomplishment. Nor do we genuinely understand the elements of activity involved in constructive tasks. Occupational therapists have talked about meaningful activity, habit training and skill acquisition for many years, but we only value them as important. With few exceptions we have not examined them scientifically.

One intriguing question for me has been the interaction between deliberate and automatic behavior, and the transition from one to the other that produces confident performance from previous uncertainty. This transition is surely what we seek in practice no matter what skill we are teaching our patients.

Beyond these fundamental questions about activity, there are clinical questions we need to ask. What activities are therapeutic, and for whom? How do we go about using them effectively? Which ones should be studied in school, etc.?

If you also think these are important issues, please let Calista and me know. We would like to think that we are not alone.

Learning to value active occupation

Originally published in *Advance for Occupational Therapy* Nov. 29, 1999

Each fall when the semester begins, my interest in inculcating in students positive notions about active occupation renews itself. Here are these cheerful faces, each person eager to become an occupational therapist, but each retaining some ideas that may actually inhibit his or her potential to succeed.

Common in our culture is the idea that 'arts and crafts' are childish and unimportant. Their artistry or occupational nature is not evident. So when we use media in labs to help students understand how activity has therapeutic value, we are faced with having to overcome ingrained ideas.

Each student who comes to study at our program must engage in a volunteer experience in an occupational therapy setting before he or she is admitted to the program. But many of the clinics are mechanistic in their approaches to therapy, and often, new students base their beliefs about occupational therapy on what they learned as volunteers. If the site did not address the occupational needs of clients, the student has no notion that active, purposeful, meaningful occupation is what makes occupational therapy work.

And at the same time that we as faculty are trying to establish fundamental ideas about meaningful occupation, these students are being heavily exposed to the sciences, which are highly regarded by much of society. Someone other than occupational therapists generally teach these sciences, so their relationship to occupational pursuits is apt to be absent. This disparity in the focus of coursework sets up a dichotomy that tends to influence choices students must make in their own occupational pursuits. Their choices shape their roles as students, and ultimately their beliefs and actions as therapists.

By way of example, due to the intensity of the curriculum, students are forced to prioritize assignments in order to manage their time. Quite naturally, many students choose the sciences and spend a great deal of time memorizing origins and insertions, organ functions, developmental sequences and learning theories. Consequently, assignments related to media often take second place. Yet the media we use are occupational tasks, and learning to do these tasks with the guidance faculty provides, clearly teaches the students fundamental ideas about occupation that they need to form their professional identity. So how to strengthen students' beliefs about the importance of activity becomes the challenge for the occupational therapy educator.

In this program we start with the Fidler Laboratory, in which students do several different activities. Here they begin to learn that human beings are unique, that activities have powerful effects and that they can be manipulated to influence a variety of factors. Students face their feelings about doing 'refrigerator art', or what they consider its equivalent, in a costly education program, and we begin to shape their pride in the power and value of occupation.

From this beginning, students are then exposed to a series of occupations from a historical, anthropological perspective, sequencing from 'clay to computers'.

Concurrent with this experiential learning, our students are exposed to lectures on the philosophic and historical origins of the profession, connecting the laboratory learning to the conceptual learning. Dewey's views of 'learning through doing' form the basis for understanding the process of occupational genesis. Lectures connect these ideas to the science learning that is also taking place.

Development, evolution, adaptation and grading are conceptually allied, and then the students explore these alliances through experiences and associated readings. But the most important feature of all in developing students' positive attitudes toward active occupation is the attitude held by the faculty. If teachers value occupation, students are apt to learn more about it. If faculty does not value occupation, students certainly will not. At our school, the faculty tends to show up to participate in the media labs even if it isn't part of their teaching load! So the message is sent and received. Here, we want occupational therapists to become committed to lifelong learning in active occupation as a professional tool. They see that their educators believe and act on it too.

Where have all the trained occupational therapists gone?

Originally published in *Advance for Occupational Therapy* Aug. 10, 1998

It has been extremely interesting to follow the dialogue in the Occup-ther list-serve recently. What began as a discussion of the problems occupational therapists have had in keeping ADL as their special 'turf' has turned into a discussion of how occupational therapists have to change in order to keep their practices viable.

And what changes must take place? One of the suggestions Noel Levan proposes, giving attribution to Michael Pizzi, is a fantasy that he has. 'I'd love to enter a "common" occupational therapy clinic/treatment space on a Sunday evening. I would remove all of the cones, pulleys, thera-anything, shoulder wheels, Herring arm tracks, etc.' The insinuation is that on Monday, occupational therapists would be forced to use all manner of occupational tools and materials in creative ways.

Money and recognition have been the catalysts for the current concern, as embattled occupational therapists bristle at seeing other professions lay claim to what occupational therapists consider their area of practice. Yet occupational therapists have themselves adopted the skills that rightly belong to other professions, while at the same time allowing their own valuable skills to dissipate. By enabling people to assume their roles in society through active occupation training, we employ our economic viability; unfortunately, we are not articulating it so that everyone can understand it. We also have neglected to examine and quantify the cost-effectiveness of our practice.

Occupational therapists have believed it is cost effective to return people to their highest levels of functioning since we first set up shop; now, with concern for finances having overtaken the health care arena, being 'cost effective' is the trait that everyone wants to emulate.

It is not too late to make our case, but it requires that we change our practices. What will happen when we remove those pegs and cones during the night? Unfortunately, all too few therapists have the skills in the use of tools and materials that might replace the hated items.

Some of the list-serve discussants argue for replacing the evil objects with leatherwork tools, decks of cards, flour and yeast and the like. But the suggestions are narrowly framed. The rationale behind these modalities is assumed to be understood – that is, any occupational therapist could appropriately deliver them. Yet, all too many occupational therapists could not. They are ill equipped to practice without the use of 'standardized' tools. In fact, the profession's focus on standardization has led us to this dilemma. Occupation is not a standardized phenomenon. To expect occupational therapy to operate in a standardized way is misinformed. Rather, it operates on a comprehensive understanding of the complexity and uniqueness of individuals. The ability to use a broad variety of tools and materials to help patients develop their personal roles is what has made occupational therapy successful in meeting people's needs.

One correspondent questions, 'How did we get this way?' A number of answers are put forth in terms of the history of medical practice. However, for occupational therapists, the answer lies in education as well as in the clinics. One by one, schools have dropped from their curricula courses that teach students the manipulative and analytic skills they need. If you don't know how to do it, you aren't going to use it.

Many of the ideas the list-serve communicates are excellent. They are not enough, but they are a start. The consensus exhibited in the dialogue is the best indication that I have seen in years that we have a problem, and that we have the wherewithal to solve it. Our best heads must come together and find solutions, and find ways to explain our solutions, before we are so out of touch that we no longer have people who think outside the box.

Susan Berres offered one of the best suggestions when she described a German clinic where the occupational therapists 'didn't have any treatment space at all – we were everywhere. We had access to a workroom full of woodworking tools; gardening supplies; paint, paper, pencils, shovels, brooms, buckets, etc., etc. And of course, there were the patient rooms themselves, full of windows to be washed, sinks to clean, socks to rinse out, beds to be made, shelves to be organized, and so on.'

If you think this cannot happen in the US, think again. One requirement that I insisted on for my practice was that we had no delegated occupational therapy room, just a closet to keep our things. That way, no one could tell us we were in someone else's space. All space was occupational therapy space, if it was where patients were. And it was clear to everyone in the facility that we had the skills necessary to function in every quarter. Furthermore, everyone understood what we could do with patients, and the referrals came from every source.

We must come to value once more the mundane and diverse activities in which human beings engage in their lives, and learn to use them to enhance our patients' abilities to function.

Writing and teaching about activity

Published in *Advance for Occupational Therapy* April 20, 1998

For too long, those of us who make note of these things have observed a decline in the use of therapeutic activity. All occupational therapy schools once included active, purposeful occupation in curricula that remained there until the mid 1960s when, due in part to expanding educational demands, a reorganization of many curricula began to take place.

The easiest courses to cut were the craft courses. After all, all occupational therapy applicants had crafts backgrounds or they would not have been interested in occupational therapy. One by one the courses were deleted and replaced by intense scientific and theoretical courses. At some schools, crafts were eliminated entirely, the expectation being that students and therapists would gain these skills on their own.

Crafts began to assume a lesser role in the clinic largely because the newest therapists had few skills, and still worse, did not understand activity and could not articulate or justify its use. But some of us – the ones who valued activity and could use it therapeutically – remained. Perhaps, we pondered, we could toss this diminishing phenomenon around and increase the appropriate use of active occupation as a tool of practice.

Talking and writing about activity began to consume me, and, I had been engaging in the process of establishing both occupational therapy and occupational therapy assistant programs at Touro College in Manhattan. Needless to say, my interests in activities consumed a bit of my time there as well. I was reaching therapists through the written word and students in the classroom and laboratory. My premise was 'if one teaches students to use activities appropriately, then they will use activities in the clinic'. Certainly, it is clear that without this teaching, students would be void of this ability.

I rely on a conceptual foundation I call 'occupational genesis' for the courses I teach and the writing I do. It has enabled me to share my ideas with greater clarity. Some of you are kind enough to let me know what you think of those ideas, as well as correspond on e-mail. Occupational genesis is based on recognition of the relationship between the mind and body of each individual, the tangible world in which he/she lives, works and plays, and the social environment which structures the roles and responsibilities of each. I call these three elements the egocentric (mind/body), exocentric (time/space), and consensual (social/cultural) realms. Furthermore, a developmental theme pervades these relationships, and it is this development that occupational therapy practitioners seek to facilitate.

Now that two groups of fledglings are about to complete their occupational therapy educations, I have begun to reap some interesting rewards. The phone has begun to ring with feedback from clinical supervisors. Charlotte Weiss called me the other day and said, 'I don't know what you are doing, but keep it up. Your students not only know how to do activities, they can apply them. And by the way, I cut out your articles and hang them up for the younger therapists to read.' This is from a clinician who is working in an environment that falls within the restrictions of modern health care reimbursement constraints.

Comments like that are always welcome, needless to say. But of greater interest to me are the comments I have been getting from the students, both OTRs and OTAs. It is really clear to them when they see good occupational therapy being delivered. They are excellent judges of the therapists whom they observe. And their comments are not based on whether they personally like or dislike someone, but on whether the therapy they see being delivered represents our profession appropriately. The students are interested in whether therapists can use their therapeutic tools to elicit growth in their patients, a growth based on the integration of the patient, the environment and the life he or she will need to lead.

Soon I will be teaching a capstone course to the occupational therapy students called 'Advanced Analysis and Synthesis of Activity'. Each of the students will strive to learn something he or she has always wanted to learn, in hopes of recognizing how meaningful activity consumes one and brings wellness. Now all that is left is to watch them enter the profession, deliver authentic occupational therapy and be role models for competent practice.

Moving into the occupation mode

Originally published in *Advance for Occupational Therapy* July 3, 2000

Something remarkable seems to happen in the minds of students as they move from their applicant status through their student role toward assuming their identity as occupational therapists. Maybe it's because they have to explain their profession to others so often. Certainly it happens as part of the educational process. If educators have done their jobs well, students learn to use their tools of occupation as tools of therapy. However, learning to value occupation is a necessary part of learning to use it therapeutically.

Students in our classes are required to learn to use every manner of occupation from 'clay to computers' as they proceed through the curriculum. If students can get past their own initial doubts about how these things work in a medical environment, they can learn to accept the value of meaningful activity as a practice tool. Our students are paying considerable sums of money to attend these classes (a fact regularly brought home to them by parents or spouses when the students bring home their 'refrigerator art' from graduate school).

Our first laboratory, the Fidler Activity Lab, includes finger paint and magazine cutouts for collage. The second lab deals with clay. The most important aspect of both those labs, aside from the recognizable therapeutic qualities students discern from analyzing their attendant activities, is that the door is always open to discussing feelings. By drawing out their own feelings of uncertainty or perhaps inadequacy at this early stage of their occupational therapy education, we begin work on this festering issue immediately, allowing us to help students learn the worth of these activities so that they can use them in practice. We are fortunate to have a faculty dedicated to active occupation in their work and personal lives, so we have role models for students to emulate. Even those of the faculty for whom the media labs are not assigned classes tend to show up periodically because they find the class so much fun and a great opportunity to extend the topics of their own lectures in a meaningful environment.

I like to watch the students grow in their skills and in their confidence in their ability to incorporate meaningful activity into therapeutic application. Students are always reporting how they used this or that activity in fieldwork. But they also report how often they encounter uncertainty from clinicians during their fieldwork experiences. By going back and forth from clinic to class, sharing their ideas and experiences, these students reinforce their learning and their beliefs in the value of meaningful activity. Of course I revel in their various tales, but sometimes an event occurs that is particularly memorable and warrants repeating.

One of our graduating students, Jen D'Aloia, stopped by at the end of the day from her fieldwork site to tell us about a job she had just accepted, and the therapeutic event in which she had participated. Jen had been doing her fieldwork at the hospital where two Seton Hall students remain hospitalized following the dormitory fire here in January that killed three freshmen. She had spent a good deal of time on the burn unit, where one of the young men had burns that severely restricted his chest, neck and arm movements.

The young man's birthday came around, and a celebration was in order. Along with the standard birthday cake and songs, our student had another idea. She brought a piñata to the hospital, hung it up and presented the young man with a bat. Without another word, he swung the bat at the piñata with all the force he could muster, using muscles and joints he had not used since January. Tears, laughter and excitement ensued among those watching. The activity had released the inhibitions the young man had, enabling him to move despite pain and fear.

As it happened, representatives of the hospital's public relations department were on hand taking photos. They cheered as well, but said, 'Physical therapy is great!' Our student boldly replied, 'That's not physical therapy, it's occupational therapy'. She knew the difference and was proud. It was the occupational therapy student who had recognized the potential value of this activity for our young man, and it was she who confidently took it upon herself to bring the piñata to the hospital because she recognized its value as a therapeutic tool.

Of course the job she was offered was at that same hospital. They are hiring a great occupational therapist!

Where do we go from here?

Originally published in *Advance for Occupational Therapy* Nov. 6, 2000

Lots of changes have been taking place in the profession over the past several years. We have moved the educational process to the masters degree as a minimum entry level for the profession. Now we are beginning the process of replacing Uniform Terminology with a document that in its draft form is called a Framework for Occupational Therapy Practice, a document that focuses heavily on occupation as a tool for health and practice [*in the United States – EBB*].

We hear more and more about occupation as a foundation for practice, but at the same time we are being faced with proposed changes in physical therapy and other licensure laws that potentially impact our practice. Job security is uncertain as the political process unfolds, and health care financing is caught up in that process.

On the other hand, as more traditional markets dry up, occupational therapists are reaching out into the community and developing new practice areas. More therapists are entering private practice, and fewer are working in the medical arena. Change is clearly upon us.

So where do we go from here? And how do we get there?

Seton Hall University, where I work, is taking a new approach to the post-professional education of occupational therapists. In addition to its professional programs in a variety of health fields, the School of Graduate Medical Education at Seton Hall currently offers a PhD in Health Sciences. A core set of courses in research and philosophy characterizes this interdisciplinary degree program, but students can elect an area of specialization to meet their own needs. Within this PhD program, there are several specialization tracks available. These include movement science, speech and language pathology, and health professions leadership. A new track is scheduled to join these in January. [*While the program received all necessary institutional approvals at the time this article was originally written, it was withdrawn by SHU administration in the spring of 2001 as part of a school-wide policy decision – EBB.*] The focus of study of this new program is Occupational Technology.

The curriculum in Occupational Technology is designed to examine in depth the nature of occupation's influence on health through the use of technology, and technology's influence on occupation and health. The approach to the study of occupation and technology is both modern and historical, recognizing that human endeavor has a long history dating back to earliest peoples, and is leading to a future yet unknown.

This program was designed by occupational therapists and is anticipated to attract occupational therapists and perhaps those with allied interests, so they can prepare for the uncertain future which we all face.

Seton Hall University is an ideal venue for this program. It has been described as the #1 wired Catholic university in the country and is widely recognized in the broader academic community for its technological proficiency, having received national awards in this area.

Occupational therapists have valued technology and utilized it in sophisticated ways from the outset of the profession in 1917. And they have kept abreast of technological gains as they have developed. All of the media we have used traditionally are forms of technology.

But we did not stop at crafts. We continued to develop our expertise in electronic technology as well, adapting these media for patients' use. Adaptive technology, assistive technology, information technology and instructional technology all are within the purview of occupational therapy. We use each of these methods to aid patients in performing life tasks. Having expertise in these areas is vital to our further growth as a profession, as society comes to depend more heavily on technology for all activities.

As we move forward in a changing society, we must become recognized experts in our pursuits. To do so, doctoral education suitable to the needs of occupational therapists must be made available. We need doctorally prepared educators and researchers to teach our students and validate our beliefs.

Primary among these beliefs is our conviction that active occupation is fundamental to health and development. We need the tools to examine these ideas. Doctoral education will provide these tools, and will provide the profession with needed experts who are capable of addressing these issues. Public recognition of that expertise is advanced by providing evidence in the form of doctoral degrees.

Of great concern in the education of occupational therapists is their ability to study in areas that permit them to hold with their beliefs. In the past, some doctoral education has drawn occupational therapists away from their core beliefs and towards a belief system that may be in conflict. Consequently, we need doctoral programs that are consistent with occupational therapy beliefs, or the ideas we hold dear will not be examined with the full support they deserve.

Occupational Technology is such a program. It will provide a framework for studying that is compatible with what occupation therapists believe: active occupation is an evolutional developmental and adaptive phenomenon that contributes to the health of the individual and the community. Recognizing the impact of technology on that phenomenon is vital if we are to stay current in a changing world.

Being able to think deep thoughts, raise important issues and answer telling questions will bring us to a new level of understanding and contribution. And with that understanding, we will further contribute to the profession and to society. Wish us luck!

Media education based on the philosophy of pragmatism

Originally published in *American Journal of Occupational Therapy*, July 1989, 43(7): 25–8

Abstract

The responsibility for crafts instruction at New York University was transferred recently from the Art Department to the Department of Occupational Therapy, where a new model of media education has been developed. This change resulted from the difficulties students and faculty experienced in integrating craft activities with occupational therapy's conceptual foundations and the realities of practice. These problems are not unique to this university but are common throughout our profession. This paper will discuss these problems and an attempt at their solution by outlining a model for media education based on historical and philosophical concepts pertinent to the profession. This model demonstrates the academic justification for the development and presentation of media education courses by occupational therapy faculty.

When the profession of occupational therapy originated, crafts were used to a greater extent than they customarily are used today. Modern occupational therapy education reflects this de-emphasis on crafts. The number of hours educators spend teaching crafts today is markedly reduced. Yet, because practice continues to use such activities, occupational therapy educators remain concerned with selecting appropriate methods for crafts instruction.

Until recently at New York University, occupational therapy students were taught crafts under the aegis of the Art Department. The influence of the art teachers on students, along with the small number of hours spent studying crafts, tended to separate the concepts underlying the use of crafts as a therapeutic tool from the mastery of crafts techniques. As a result, crafts instruction proved problematic, necessitating repeated faculty intervention over an 8-year period to refine course content so that it might better meet the needs of occupational therapy students (Donahue, personal communication, October 1987). Because faculty members who were not occupational therapists taught these courses, the foundational principles of the profession were not well integrated with the material presented in the crafts courses. In addition, it was extremely difficult to establish the relevance of craft activities in relation to other activities such as activities of daily living or computer fluency. Consequently, crafts became trivialized and students experienced some feelings of fragmentation; many had difficulty understanding how crafts related to other aspects of the profession, particularly because some clinical sites used crafts very little or not at all. Although the theoretical aspects of activity and occupation were addressed elsewhere in the curriculum, the relevance of crafts was not well understood by students.

Contributing to these feelings of fragmentation was the fact that crafts courses were taught within a department whose philosophy was built on aesthetics, a philosophy that differs from and is inconsistent with occupational therapy's philosophy of active occupation. Measures taken to synthesize concepts of activity with their instruction were unsuccessful because faculty members did not sufficiently identify and emphasize the philosophical differences of the two departments.

Historically, crafts at New York University had been taught within the Industrial Arts Department. When the Occupational Therapy Department was established in 1942, the concepts underlying study within that department were consistent with those of the Industrial Arts Department, stemming from the belief that active occupation contributes to learning in all human beings. Eventually, due to internal organizational changes, the responsibility for the crafts courses was transferred from the Industrial

Arts Department to the Art Department, where principles of aesthetics are premier. However valuable they may be, these principles are not characteristic of occupational therapy. Rather, performance itself and its implications for learning and development are the predominant principles of occupational therapy. This inconsistency in focus was one of the reasons that occupational therapy students repeatedly questioned the need to study crafts in general and to take the courses offered through the Art Department specifically. Due to this discrepancy, implications for occupational therapy media education began to emerge.

Despite the occupational therapy faculty's desire and prolonged efforts to rectify the educational problem, no arguments had proven successful in convincing university officials that these courses could best be taught by the Department of Occupational Therapy. Yet, the inconsistencies between departmental philosophies had implications for education; therefore, if articulated clearly, they could serve as the basis for an argument that would be recognized by the academic community. If inconsistent philosophical messages contributed to the problems in the crafts courses, perhaps the courses needed to be totally restructured so that they clearly reflected the appropriate educational philosophy. This would necessitate shifting the responsibility for the courses to a department that believes that the concepts of active occupation are foremost.

The questions that students expressed are not exclusive to them. Many therapists are also uncertain about why crafts were traditionally used in practice, and why they continue to be taught. On the other hand, many therapists retain a strong commitment to the use of crafts in education and practice. However, some are inadequately prepared to articulate their reasons for this commitment, partly because they were never taught many of the concepts that contributed to our profession's adoption of active occupation as a therapeutic tool.

Several people (Diasio, 1968; Dunning, 1973; Laurencelle, 1968; Owen, 1968; Yerxa, 1967) have discussed the need for our profession to identify its philosophy in an attempt to answer questions the profession has about itself. In response, the Representative Assembly of the American Occupational Therapy Association (AOTA) adopted Resolution C, which articulates the Philosophical Base of Occupational Therapy (AOTA, 1979b, p. 785). Further research identified other philosophical sources than those investigated at that time (Breines, 1986a).

Occupational therapy's history contains two related philosophical themes that were concurrently advanced by many of the same people. One was pragmatism, the American philosophy that emphasized activity and adaptation; the other was the arts and crafts movement, a philosophy of British origin that emphasized the amelioration of the unhealthy influences of industrialization (Breines, 1986a; Levine, 1987). Both philosophies were concerned with creating a healthy society by addressing the meaning of activity in human lives.

The problem with terms such as *health* and *activity* is that their significance is apt to be lost. That is what occurred with crafts. Crafts remained a tool of practice, but without a comprehensive rationale it was difficult to justify their use. Consequently, crafts were retained in the educational curriculum but were unconnected to their philosophical underpinnings. To rectify this, the faculty at New York University examined occupational therapy's philosophy and its implications for the instruction of students in the value of activity in health and development; they then developed courses integrating the study of crafts with these philosophical foundations.

Philosophy of pragmatism for occupation and education

John Dewey (1916), the education philosopher, applied the principles of pragmatism to education. He concluded that learning recapitulates humanity's past experience, and is best synthesized through active experience. To demonstrate these concepts, he designed a laboratory school at the University of Chicago that was based on these principles (Mayhew and Edwards, 1936). His students learned by engaging in tasks performed by increasingly complex cultures. As the students advanced in grade, these tasks, and the knowledge required to perform them, became more complex. For example, in early grades students studied a hunter-gatherer society; in later grades they studied an agrarian society; and still later they studied more complex societies. Students learned the tasks of living, or occupations, that permitted each society and its individuals to survive, thereby gaining the knowledge inherent in those tasks. Instruction focused on the interdependence of the members of a society working together in tasks of mutual benefit.

Jane Addams (1910), Dewey's neighbor at Hull House, the famous settlement house, and his colleague at the University of Chicago, was a friend and co-worker of Julia Lathrop (Addams, 1935), a founder of the first school of occupational therapy (Dunton, 1915). At Hull House, Addams and Lathrop used these same concepts to help immigrants understand the relationship between their heritage and their roles in their new society. Addams demonstrated that the hand-spindles their ancestors used for spinning made the same contribution to society as spinning wheels and the spinning machines used in the industrialized world. This analysis of activity and its grading led to the concepts of grading activity that became a part of occupational therapy. These ideas were based on a comprehensive view of heritage that was expressed in terms of activity.

Cultures develop active occupations to meet their needs. Members of society meet their needs for food, clothing, shelter, and spirituality both individually and collaboratively. Methods of communication develop that enhance this process. As children develop into adults, they acquire skills that contribute to their own needs and to those of their society, first through play (Reilly, 1974) and then through work. As societies evolve, they retain the skills of earlier cultures, adapting them in ways that permit new concepts, inventions, and environmental constraints to be synthesized with the old. Thus, tasks and skills that originally met certain needs become incorporated with new development in unique and original ways that often benefit society in new ways.

Primitive hunter-gatherer cultures, such as aborigines and the American Indians, used media and activities such as pottery, leather crafts, basketry, and totem making to meet their needs. By adapting these skills, nomadic people such as the Bedouins and the Masai, learned to herd their food supply, and create specialized clothing, shelter, and objects that could be carried from place to place. More complex cultures refined these skills. The weaving of reeds and grasses developed into the spinning of flax, fleece, and silk into thread, then into the weaving of fabric. This led to further developments in cloth construction. Drop spindles and weaving frames were developed into spinning wheels and harness looms, which brought spinning and weaving to new levels. Similar developments occurred in other media, fostered by the needs of particular societies congruent with various environmental constraints. As societies became agrarian and began to harvest food, their mobility became limited. This necessitated the creation of permanent residences, along with the development of associated knowledge and skills. With the advent of trade, refinements in mathematics and written language evolved. Technology advanced throughout the Bronze and Iron Ages and beyond. With wheels, gears, fulcrums, and levers, a science of engineering emerged. These developments led to the Industrial Revolution, with its characteristic specialization and mechanization, first with water and wind, then with steam, and then with electricity. Electricity led to electronics and the modern technologies of energy waves, chemistry, and plastics; eventually it led to the nuclear age and the space age. Over time, religious figures lost their animistic forms and were altered to human form; this led to further abstractions of god concepts, and to godless societies. All of these religious beliefs are represented in the modern world.

Tools, skills, and beliefs all develop in accordance with people's needs, as enabled or restricted by their environments (Piaget, 1979). The inventions of earlier civilizations are retained through all of these changes, altered in form and purpose, but still meaningful to society, both in their original and in their adapted dimensions. These concepts of development, evolution, and active occupation were adopted as pedagogical principles by Dewey (1916).

Teaching active occupation

Occupational therapy theory and practice advocates the use of skills, tools, and the environment in active occupation to meet humankind's needs. Therapists must be knowledgeable about these concepts and the performance of related tasks. To instruct patients in relevant activities, a therapist must (a) be skilled in the activities used in practice, (b) know the reasons they are used, and (c) use them in a culturally appropriate fashion. Because the uses of activity are broad, a comprehensive understanding of the principles that underlie the use of activity as a therapeutic tool is essential.

To address this need at New York University, a set of courses was proposed that included a spectrum of activities reflecting the developmental aspects of mankind's adaptation to the world. These courses illustrate the nature of phylogenetic and ontogenetic development. They demonstrate humans' involvement in adaptive tasks throughout their individual development and their history, into the modern era. These courses demonstrate that activity is a part of every society; that pertinent, contributing activity is healthful for individuals and for society; and that crafts are part of our profession's heritage but must be understood in terms of the skills they offer in evolution and development. This approach reveals the relationships between crafts and technology, individual tasks and group tasks, and the development of knowledge and the maturation of the individual and society.

Media courses dealing with development, evolution, and the grading of active occupations must include instruction in techniques. Consequently, New York University faculty determined that such courses should (a) provide opportunities for students to explore all sorts of activities and (b) reveal the evolutional theme of active occupation. The courses that were developed include the following selected tasks. During the first-semester course, emphasis is placed on the crafts that are commonly used in hunter-gatherer and agrarian society. Pottery making, leather crafts, and basketry are studied, followed by yarn crafts and fabric crafts. During the second-semester course, crafts of industrial and technological societies are emphasized. Printing and paper crafts, wood crafts, and metal crafts are taught, along with the use of mechanical and electrical equipment, electronics, and computers.

The relationships between these content areas are demonstrated by an emphasis on the concepts of evolution, development, grading of activities, activity analysis, activity synthesis, and implications for therapy. The learning objectives for these courses stipulate that students will come to understand the role of occupational therapy's foundational philosophy of pragmatism in the profession's theme of active occupation. Students are expected to comprehend the nature of cultural evolution and its significance in relation to active occupation in all societies. They are required to demonstrate skill in selected crafts and activities, and to understand how crafts and skills have evolved and been adapted to meet environmental and sociocultural demands, as well as the specialized needs of individuals in evolving societies. In addition, students must demonstrate skill in teaching selected crafts and activities, and must collaborate in problem-solving tasks using media to meet selected physical and psychosocial demands. The courses are designed to help students understand that activities that range from clay to computers meet life's needs in various civilizations. This approach to media education prepares students not only to use traditional crafts as therapeutic tools but also to use modern and future technologies that will be developed as humanity continues to evolve.

Conclusion

When instructed by art teachers, occupational therapy students had difficulty understanding the value of crafts as tools of practice. Once the issue was identified as a difference in philosophical orientation rather than a deficiency in educational technique, artistic expertise, or application of therapeutic principles by instructors who were artists, it was clear to the Occupational Therapy and Art Departments and to the academic administration that the curriculum needed to be altered. Changes in instructors or content, as had been attempted in the past, could not ameliorate the differences in philosophic beliefs. Rather, the courses needed to be taught as part of an integrated conceptual view of occupational therapy by qualified instructors who hold those beliefs. With the approval of the university, the Art Department willingly and generously withdrew the courses it had formerly taught, and the courses described above replaced them. These new courses are now in place; they are taught within the department of Occupational Therapy by occupational therapists. It remains only to evaluate the effects of this approach on the students' learning and satisfaction and on their ability to practice occupational therapy using purposeful activities in an integrated way.

Acknowledgments

I want to express my sincere appreciation for the generous contributions of Dr Deborah R. Labovitz, Dr Rosalie J. Miller, Dr Mary V. Donahue, Professor Karen Buckley, Professor Sharon Lefkofsky, and Professor Paula McCreedy of the Department of Occupational Therapy at New York University, in the development of these courses and the writing of this paper.

Occupational therapy education in a technological world

Originally published in *American Journal of Occupational Therapy* July/Aug. 2002, 56(4): 467–8

Curricula across the country are grappling with how to teach technology in occupational therapy professional education programs. Although the *Standards for an Accredited Education Program for the Occupational Therapist* (Accreditation Council of Occupational Therapy Education, 1999) stipulate the inclusion of technology content, this requirement does not provide guidelines of what to include or a framework for pedagogy. Because technology includes both low-tech adaptations and high-tech electronic solutions (Moyers, 1999), students must learn adaptive technologies, assistive technologies, telecommunications, and data management in order to be adequately prepared. Additionally, students must be prepared for other technological advances to meet future challenges as therapists.

Technology is linked to occupational therapy practice through occupation. This link helps to guide a modern curriculum. The profession recognizes that occupational therapy practice revolves around the everyday occupations and roles of clients (Christiansen and Baum, 1997). Social and cultural norms, including the use of technology, often dictate those occupations. Over the years, technology has become essential to occupational therapy practice and in the preparation of future therapists.

Technology and occupational therapy

Occupational therapists have been writing about computers and technology for decades (Angelo and Smith, 1993). In 1983, the Occupational Therapy Computer Club first met in Portland, Oregon, and began a grassroots journal (e.g. Breines, 1985). From then on, therapists have considered curriculum issues for technology learning (Angelo, 1997; Angelo, Buning, Schmeler and Doster, 1997; Anson, 1997; Breines, 1985; Hammel and Luebben, 1996; Kanny, Anson and Smith, 1991). However, the technological interests that guided the profession from its outset are rarely if ever cited and have seemed to be taken for granted. The foundational technical skills in which occupational therapists have customarily been trained has not yet been well integrated into the learning of modern technology-based skills.

History of technology in occupational therapy

Occupational therapists have always been technologists, adapting themselves and their clients to the environments in which they live and work. At the outset of the profession, societies worldwide were transitioning from agriculture to industry. The notions of activity analysis and adaptation helped to define occupational therapy and remain important as this process results in the continuous updating of practice (Breines, 1986a; Gilbreth, 1911). To prepare therapists to facilitate healthful adaptation within any changing era, students are taught to use familiar tools and materials, learning handcrafts or industrial activities as contextually appropriate (Breines, 1995).

Today, people use computer-operated devices in their work, schools, supermarkets, banks, transportation and leisure. What is not clear, however, is which technology instruction should be included within an occupational therapy curriculum (Hammel and Angelo, 1996; Hammel and Smith, 1996).

An integrated technology curriculum for occupational therapy education

Seton Hall University (SHU) is recognized nationally for its high level of expertise in technology as a learning tool (Lowe, 1999; Sheeran, 2001; Winters, 1998; Yahoo Internet Life, 2002). Within this academic environment, the occupational therapy program has created a graded technology curriculum. Incoming students receive laptop computers through a ubiquitous computing program ('Wired for Success', 1999). Before the first semester begins, students attend a workshop to introduce them to the computer so that they can participate in learning assignments that grow in complexity throughout the 3 years of the program. Numerous optional campus-wide workshops teach various skills for computer use, making it possible for students to approach computer learning as an individualized skill set. Given the varied preparation with which students enter graduate education, this self-directed approach works well. All students receive standard software preloaded onto their computers. The software bundle includes WordPerfect, Excel, PowerPoint, Front Page, and Publisher[1]; Statistical Package for the Social Sciences (SPSS)[2]; Netscape Communicator[3]; Internet Explorer[4]; and Blackboard[5].

The curriculum sequence leads students as they build their technology skills. During the first semester, students learn that all manual activities are technological and that societies develop through the integration of technology. Based on a sociological model grounded in the philosophy of pragmatism (Breines, 1986a, 1989b; Dewey, 1916; Mayhew and Edwards, 1936), they begin to develop skill in tool use. They learn handcrafts, including clay, basketry, leather and yarn, while examining the evolution of occupations and cultures. They visit the American Museum of Natural History in New York City where they view changes in occupational technology (Breines, 2001; Breines, Picard, Torcivia and Avi-Itzhak, in press).

As the program evolves, students use the computer as a tool for increasingly challenging assignments. Initially, they respond by e-mail to assigned questions. Then they perform activity analyses that require them to share document attachments of boilerplate forms. All assignments must be word processed using the Publication Manual of the American Psychological Association (APA, 2001), which can be accessed through the SHU library home page. Students are introduced to Blackboard, a Web-based education platform, interview a virtual visitor to the classroom through wireless technology accessed with their laptops, and participate in synchronous and asynchronous electronic class discussions.

In the second year, students acquire skills in industrial activities that include woodworking, stenciling, metal and plastic crafts, and basic wiring, analyzing these activities while examining their relevance for industrial societies and the modern workforce. They visit workers on and off campus, looking at their use of high-tech and low-tech tools while analyzing the impact of work on health. They complete a course in splinting, using low-temperature thermoplastics and wiring techniques. They prepare PowerPoint presentations, use the Internet as a research tool, and learn to recognize the limitations of Web-based research.

During the third year of the program, students' modern technology education intensifies. They visit hardware purveyors, such as Home Depot[6] or Radio Shack[7], to identify source materials. They collaborate to assemble a Web-based document on leisure activity while individual students create Web pages. Students learn about electricity and the basic construction and use of adaptive switches. They learn the mechanical aspects of computer hardware, view the interior of computers, and practice installing internal and external mechanisms. They study adaptive technologies and apply their uses in case simulations and clinical situations. To build their skills as educated consumers, students identify vendors and invite them to present various aspects of assistive technology, ranging from seating systems to voice-activated software and environmental controls. They explore the uses of technology in public systems and private enterprises. For advanced activity analysis exercises, students analyze software and hardware. In the curriculum's management course, students create promotional materials, such as business cards, brochures, and fliers, with creativity software. They use the scanner to transfer copy and designs, develop budgets with Excel, and use SPSS for data management in the research courses.

Discoveries

Because technology changes rapidly, its availability to the curriculum has changed since its inception. Originally, SHU's Teaching, Learning and Technology Center supported a Learning Space platform, which advanced to Blackboard after a trial period. Although faculty members required retraining and reconfiguration of their course materials, moving to wireless computing enhanced what we were able to introduce in class. Students' computers no longer needed to be plugged to a cable.

Some of the most inexpensive instructional software has been found in the sales buckets at Staples[8] and Marshalls[9]. We were able to purchase a wide variety of games and other software with this method for students to perform activity analyses. One of these purchases assists students with architectural design layouts when studying accessibility issues. We also found that vendors were generally open to providing equipment demonstrations, which saved substantially on purchasing costly equipment and avoided concerns about obsolescence. This strategy has been helpful for both information technology and assistive technology instruction.

Overall, we discovered that the students themselves serve as an exceptional technology resource. Each subsequent class brings greater technology skill than the one preceding it, mirroring society's advances. Students are eager to share what they know and bring one another along in their competencies.

Summary

As occupational therapy curricula prepare students to meet the needs of clients living in a technological world, at SHU we have chosen to emphasize professional survival and practice in a technology learning context. The curriculum is guided throughout by the pedagogy of learning through doing (Dewey, 1916), using technology-based learning that increases in complexity and application as the program advances. This education results in the professional preparation of therapists who are equipped to apply their skills in the treatment of clients living in a modern world. Aspects of this approach, which ties technology to occupation, might be considered by other training programs in different settings.

Acknowledgments

I thank Elizabeth M. Torcivia, MPA, OTR, and Meryl M. Picard, MSW, OTR, for their contributions to the development of the technology aspects of the Occupational Therapy Program at Seton Hall University and for their review of this article.

Notes

1. Microsoft Corporation, One Microsoft Way, Redmond, Washington 98052-6399.
2. Statistical Package for the Social Sciences (SPSS) 233 S. Wacker Drive, Chicago, Illinois 60606
3. Netscape Communications, Inc., PO Box 7050, Mountain View, California 94039-7050
4. Microsoft Corporation, One Microsoft Way, Redmond, Washington 98052-6399.
5. Blackboard, Inc. 202-463-4860, 202-463-4863 (fax); www.blackboard.com.
6. Home Depot, 2455 Paces Ferry Road, Atlanta, Georgia 30339.
7. Radio Shack, 3DD West Third Street, Suite 14DD, Ft. Worth, Texas 76102.
8. Staples, 500 Staples Drive, Framingham, Massachusetts 01701.
9. Marshalls, 770 Cochituate Road, Framingham, Massachusetts 01701

References

Accreditation Council for Occupational Therapy Education (ACOTE) (1998) Standards for an Accredited Educational Program for the Occupational Therapist. Bethesda, MD: ACOTE, American Occupational Therapy Association.

Accreditation Council for Occupational Therapy Education (ACOTE) (1999) Standards for an Accredited Educational Program for the Occupational Therapist. American Journal of Occupational Therapy 53: 575–82.

Addams J (1910) Twenty Years at Hull House. New York: Macmillan.

Addams J (1925) Twenty Years at Hull House, with autobiographical notes, by Jane Addams. New York: Macmillan.

Addams J (1935) My Friend Julia Lathrop. New York: Macmillan.

ADVANCE Staff (1994) Occupation is work, says the public – but other activities have more meaning. ADVANCE for Occupational Therapists, May 30, 13:46.

American Museum of Natural History (2002) Hall of South American Peoples. New York.

American Occupational Therapy Association (c. 1918) Description of early curriculum. Notes of a reconstruction aide. American Occupational Therapy Association Archives, University of Texas Medical Branch, Moody Medical Library, Galveston, TX.

American Occupational Therapy Association (1979a) American Occupational Therapy Association Resolution 531. Rockville, MD: Author.

American Occupational Therapy Association (1979b) 1979 Representative Assembly – 59th Annual conference [Minutes]. American Journal of Occupational Therapy 33: 781–813.

American Psychological Association (APA) (2001) Publication Manual of the American Psychological Association, 5th edn. Washington, DC: Author.

Angelo J (1997) Assistive Technology for Rehabilitation Therapists. Philadelphia: F.A. Davis.

Angelo J, Smith RO (1993) An analysis of computer-related articles in occupational therapy periodicals. American Journal of Occupational Therapy 47: 25–9.

Angelo J, Buning ME, Schmeler M, Doster S (1997) Identifying best practice in the occupational therapy assistive technology evaluation: an analysis of three focus groups. American Journal of Occupational Therapy 51(10): 916–20.

Anson DK (1997) Alternative Computer Access: A Guide to Selection. Philadelphia: F.A. Davis.

Atkinson RD, Court RD (1998) The New Economy Index: Understanding America's Economic Transformation. Washington, DC: Progressive Policy Institute.

Ayer AJ (1968) The Origins of Pragmatism: Studies in the Philosophy of Charles Sanders Peirce and William James. San Francisco: Freeman, Cooper.

Ayres AJ (1972, 1975) Sensory Integration and Learning Disorders. Los Angeles: Western Psychological Services.

Bain BK, Leger D (1997) Assistive Technology: An Interdisciplinary approach. New York: Churchill Livingston.

Barrows M (1917) Susan E. Tracy. Maryland Psychiatric Quarterly 6 (Jan.): 59.

Barton GE (1914) Letter to Wm. R. Dunton, Jr., Clifton Springs, November 30. AOTA Archives, Moody Medical Library, University of Texas Medical Branch, Galveston, Texas.

Barton GE (c. 1914–17) Letters to William Rush Dunton, Jr. Clifton Springs, NY: AOTA Archives.

Barton GE (1919) Teaching the Sick: A Manual of Occupational Therapy and Re-education. Philadelphia: W.B. Saunders.

Batchelder H (1985) Personal discussion with reconstruction aide, Livingston, NJ, Oct. 12.

Bobath B (1979) Adult Hemiplegia: Evaluation and Treatment, 2nd edn. London: William Heinemann Medical Books Ltd.

Breines EB (1981) Perception: Its Development and Recapitulation. Lebanon, NJ: Geri-Rehab.

Breines EB (1985) IBM PC at NYU. Journal of the Occupational Therapy Computer Club 5(5).

Breines EB (1986a) Origins and Adaptations: A Philosophy of Practice. Lebanon, NJ: Geri-Rehab.

Breines EB (1986b) Pragmatism, a philosophical foundation of Occupational Therapy, 1900–1922 and 1968–1985: Implications for specialization and education. Dissertation for the degree of Ph.D. New York University.

Breines EB (1986c) A quest for certainty and identity. Keynote Address. New Jersey Occupational Therapy Association Annual Conference.

Breines EB (1987) Pragmatism as a foundation for occupational therapy curricula. American Journal of Occupational Therapy 41: 522–5.

Breines EB (1988a) The issue is: redefining professionalism for occupational therapy. American Journal of Occupational Therapy 42: 55–7.

Breines EB (1988b) The Functional Assessment Scale as an instrument for measuring changes in levels of function in nursing home residents following occupational therapy. Canadian Journal of Occupational Therapy 55: 135–40.

Breines EB (1989a) Emil G. Hirsch: a pioneer in occupational therapy. Judaism 38: 216–23.

Breines EB (1989b) Media education based on the philosophy of pragmatism. American Journal of Occupational Therapy 43: 461–4.

Breines EB (1990) Genesis of occupation: a philosophical model for therapy and theory. Australian Occupational Therapy Journal. 37: 45–9.

Breines EB (1995) Occupational Therapy Activities from Clay to Computers: Theory and Practice. Philadelphia: F.A. Davis.

Breines EB (2001) Occupational Technology. [Online]. South Orange, NJ: Seton Hall University. http://gradmeded.shu.edu/occtech.

Breines EB (2002) Technology and occupation: contemporary viewpoints – Occupational therapy education in a technological world. American Journal of Occupational Therapy 56: 467–9.

Breines EB, Picard MM, Torcivia EM, Avi-Itzhak T (in press) Occupational technology: moving the profession forward in the technological era. Occupational Therapy International.

Brunyate RW (1958) Eleanor Clarke Slagle lecture. Powerful levers in little common things. American Journal of Occupational Therapy 12: 194.

Christiansen C (1994) Classification and study in occupation: a review and discussion of taxonomies. Journal of Occupational Science 1(3): 3–21.

Christiansen C, Baum C (1997) Occupational Therapy: Enabling Function and Well-being, 2nd edn. Thorofare, NJ: Slack.

Clark F, Parham D, Carlson M et al. (1991) Occupational science: academic innovation in the service of occupational therapy's future. American Journal of Occupational Therapy 45: 300–10.

Cohen S (1983) The mental hygiene movement: the development of personality and the school: the medicalization of American education. History of Education Quarterly 23 (Summer): 123–49.

Colman W (1984) A study in educational policy setting in occupational therapy (vols. I and II). Unpublished doctoral dissertation, New York University, New York.

Cowen AD (1923) Foreword. In Memoriam: Dr. Emil G. Hirsch. Chicago Section Council of Jewish Women 4, 4, 3, Cincinnati: American Jewish Archives – Jewish Institute of Religion (AJA-JIR).

Cromwell FS (1977) Eleanor Clarke Slagle, the leader, the woman. American Journal of Occupational Therapy 31: 645–8.

Darnell JL, Heater SL (1994) The issue is: occupational therapist or activity therapist – which do you choose to be? American Journal of Occupational Therapy 48: 467–8.

Darwin CR (1859) The Origin of Species by Means of Natural Selection. New York: Macmillan-Collier Books.

Dewey J (1916) Democracy and Education: an Introduction to the Philosophy of Education. Toronto: Collier-Macmillan.

Dewey J (1929) The Quest for Certainty: a Study of the Relation of Knowledge and Action. New York: Minton, Balch.

Diasio K (1968) Psychiatric occupational therapy: search for a conceptual framework in light of psychoanalytic ego psychology and learning theory. American Journal of Occupational Therapy 22: 400–7.

Dunning RE (1973) Philosophy and occupational therapy. American Journal of Occupational Therapy 27: 18–23.

Dunton, WR (1915) Occupational therapy: a manual for nurses. Philadelphia: W.B. Saunders.

Dunton WR (c. 1916–17) Letters to Eleanor C. Slagle and Barton, Bethesda, MD: AOTA Archives.

Dunton WR (1918) Occupation aides. Maryland Psychiatric Quarterly 8: 27–8.

Dykhuizen G (1973) The Life and Mind of John Dewey. Carbondale, IL: Southern Illinois University Press.

Encyclopedia Judaica (1978) 8: columns 503–4.

English C, Kasch M, Silverman P, Walker S (1982). On the role of occupational therapists in physical disabilities. American Journal of Occupational Therapy 36: 199–202.

Fidler GS (1979) Professional or nonprofessional. In Occupational Therapy: 2001 A.D.: 31–6. Rockville, MD: American Occupational Therapy Association.

Fidler GS (1981) From crafts to competency. American Journal of Occupational Therapy 35: 567–73.

Fidler GS, Fidler JW (1978) Doing and becoming: purposeful action and self-actualization. American Journal of Occupational Therapy 32: 305–10.

Gilbreth FB (1911) Motion Study. New York: Nostrand.

GLB (1935) Reform Advocate May, 300. AJA–JIR.

Hamer DH (1984) Why do occupational therapists avoid explaining occupational therapy? Occupational Therapy Newspaper 38(2).

Hammel J, Angelo J (1996) Technology competencies for occupational therapy practitioners. Assistive Technology 8: 34–42.

Hammel J, Luebben AJ (1996) Assistive technology in occupational therapy: what is it, why do I need to know it, and what do I need to know? In J Hammel (ed.), Technology and Occupational Therapy: a Link to Function. Bethesda, MD: American Occupational Therapy Association.

Hammel J, Smith RO (1996) Assistive technology and occupational therapy: the on-ramp therapy electronic superhighway. In AOTA Self-Paced Clinical Course: Technology and Occupational Therapy: a Link to Function (Lesson 2). Bethesda, MD: American Occupational Therapy Association.

Hinojosa J, Sabari J, Rosenfeld MS (1983) Purposeful activities. AOTA Representative Assembly.

Hirsch DE (1968) Rabbi Emil Hirsch, Reform Advocate. Chicago: Whitehall.

Hirsch EG (1892) Laureate oration delivered at the commencement exercises of the Hebrew Union College. Proceedings of the Board of Governors of the Union of American Hebrew Congregations. 1891–1897, IV, 2951. AJA–JIR.

Hofstadter D (1979) Godel, Escher and Bach: the Eternal Golden Braid. New York: Basic Books.

Hopkins HL, Smith HP (1983) Willard & Spackman's Occupational Therapy. Philadelphia: Lippincott.

Huss AJ (1981) From kinesiology to adaptation. American Journal of Occupational Therapy 35: 574–80.

Jacobs K, Bettencourt CM (1995) Ergonomics for Therapists. Newton, MA: Butterworth-Heinemann.

Johnson H (1996) Osler's Web: Inside the Labyrinth of the Chronic Fatigue Syndrome Epidemic. New York: Crown.

Jung C (1964) Man and His Symbols. Garden City, NY: Doubleday.

Kanny EM, Anson DK, Smith RO (1991) Brief: a survey of technology education in entry level curricula. Quantity, quality and barriers. Occupational Therapy Journal of Research 11: 311–19.

Katz N (1985) Occupational therapy's domain of concern: reconsidered. American Journal of Occupational Therapy 39: 518–24.

Kidner TB (c. 1917) Letters to William Rush Dunton, Jr. Bethesda, MD AOTA Archives.

Kielhofner G (1982) A heritage of activity: development of theory. American Journal of Occupational Therapy 36: 723-30.

Kielhofner G, Burke JP (1980) A model of human occupation, Part 1: Conceptual framework and content. American Journal of Occupational Therapy 34: 572–81.

Kuhn T (1970) The Structure of Scientific Revolutions, 2nd edn. Chicago: University of Chicago Press.

Laurencelle P (1968) Facio, ergo cogito, ergo sum: some classical antecedents to a theory of occupational therapy. American Journal of Occupational Therapy 22: 275–7.

Levine RE (1987) Looking back – the influence of the arts-and-crafts movement of the professional status of occupational therapy. American Journal of Occupational Therapy 41: 248–54.

Licht S (1967) The founding and founders of the American Occupational Therapy Association. American Journal of Occupational Therapy 21: 269.

Lidz T (1985) Adolf Meyer and the development of American psychiatry. In KD Serrett (ed.), Philosophical and Historical Roots of Occupational Therapy. New York: Haworth.
Lindquist JE, Mack W, Parham LD (1982a) A synthesis of occupational behaviour and sensory integration concepts in theory and practice, Part 1, Theory and practice. American Journal of Occupational Therapy 36: 365–74.
Lindquist JE, Mack W, Parham LD (1982b) A synthesis of occupational behaviour and sensory integration concepts in theory and practice, Part 2. American Journal of Occupational Therapy 36: 433–7.
Llorens L (1979) Sequential care record. Paper presented at AOTA Annual Conference.
Llorens L (1980) Occupational therapy sequential client care record manual. Laurel, MD: Ramsco Publishing Company.
Lowe FH (1999) Ivy-covered web sites. Chicago Sun-Times, 3 Aug. 1999: 3.
Mann WC, Lane JP (1995) Assistive technology for persons with disabilities, 2nd edn. Bethesda, MD: American Occupational Therapy Association.
Marmer L (1994) No longer 'craft ladies', who are we now? ADVANCE for Occupational Therapists, May 30: 12.
Mayhew KC, Edwards AC (1936) The Dewey School: the Lab School of the University of Chicago, 1896–1903. New York: Appleton-Century.
Mead GH (1932) Philosophy of the Present. A.E. Murphy (ed.). Chicago: Open Court.
Mead GH (1938) Philosophy of the Act. Chicago: University of Chicago Press.
Meyer A (1913) Plans for work in the Phipps Psychiatric Clinic. Modern Hospital 1: 69–70.
Meyer A (1922) The philosophy of occupation therapy. Archives of Occupational Therapy (retitled Occupational Therapy & Rehabilitation) 1: 1–10.
Meyer A (1950–52) The Collected Papers of Adolf Meyer. EE Winters (ed.). Baltimore: Johns Hopkins Press.
Mills CW (1964) Sociology and Pragmatism: the Higher Learning in America. New York: Oxford University Press.
Molleson T (1994) The eloquent bones of Abu Hyreyra. Scientific American 118: 71–6.
Mosey AC (1970) Three Frames of Reference for Mental Health. New York: Slack.
Mosey AC (1981) Occupational Therapy: Configuration of a Profession. New York: Raven Press.
Mosey AC (1985) Eleanor Clarke Slagle Lecture, 1985: a monistic or a pluralistic approach to professional identity? American Journal of Occupational Therapy 39: 504–9.
Moyers PA (1999) The guide to occupational therapy practice. American Journal of Occupational Therapy 53: 247–89.
Nelson DL (1988) Occupation: form and performance. Americal Journal of Occupational Therapy 42: 633–41.
New Britannica/Webster Dictionary and Reference Guide (1981) Chicago: Encyclopedia Britannica, Inc.
New York Times (2000a) 9 Jan. Classified advertisements.
New York Times (2000b) 11 Jan. AOL/Times Warner.
Owen CM (1968) An analysis of the philosophy of occupational therapy. American Journal of Occupational Therapy 22: 502–5.
Piaget J (1979) Behavior and Evolution. D Nicholson-Smith (trans.). New York: Pantheon.
Post KM (1996) Where technology and occupational therapy meet: the past and the future. In J Hammel (ed.), Technology and Occupational Therapy: A Link to Function. Bethesda, MD: American Occupational Therapy Association.
Reilly M (ed.) (1974) Play as Exploratory Learning. Beverly Hills, CA: Sage Publications.

Rood A (1962) The use of sensory receptors to activate, facilitate, and inhibit motor response, autonomic and somatic in developmental sequence. In C Sattley (ed.), Approaches to the Treatment of Patients with Neuromuscular Dysfunction (Study Course VI: Third International Congress World Federation of Occupational Therapists, 1962). Dubuque, IA: Brown.

Rorty R (1982) Consequences of pragmatism (Essays: 1972–1980). Minneapolis: University of Minneapolis Press.

Sachs D (1988) The perceptions of caring held by female occupational therapists: implications for professional role and identity. Unpublished doctoral dissertation. New York University, New York.

Schkade JK, Schultz C (1992) Occupational adaptation: toward a holistic approach for contemporary practice, part 1. American Journal of Occupational Therapy 46: 829–37.

Schultz C, Schkade JK (1992) Occupational adaptation: toward a holistic approach for contemporary practice, part 2. American Journal of Occupational Therapy 46: 917–25.

Serrett KD (1985a) Another look at occupational therapy's history: paradigm or pair of hands? Occupational Therapy in Mental Health 5: 1–31.

Serrett KD (1985b) Eleanor Clarke Slagle: founder and leader in occupational therapy. Occupational Therapy in Mental Health 5: 101–8.

Serrett KD (ed.) (1985c) Philosophical and Historical Roots of Occupational Therapy. New York: Haworth Press.

Shanzel L (2000) Personal communication.

Sheeran R (2001) Beyond the first five years: lessons learned in transforming teaching and learning. EDUCAUSE Review.

Shilts R (1987) And the Band Played On: Politics, People and the AIDS Epidemic. New York: St Martin's Press.

Slagle EC (1914) History of the development of occupation for the insane. Maryland Psychiatric Quarterly 4: 14–20.

Slagle EC (c. 1916–17) Letters to William Dunton, Jr. Bethesda, MD. AOTA Archives.

Slagle EC (c. 1917). Letter to W.R. Dunton, Jr., Chicago. AOTA Archives, Moody Medical Library, University of Texas Medical Branch, Galveston, Texas.

Smith JE (1978) Purpose and Thought: the Meaning of Pragmatism. New Haven: Yale University Press.

Smith RO, Hammel J, Rein J, Anson D (1992) Technology: an occupational therapy treatment modality. OT Week, 5 March: 16–19.

Starr P (1982) The Social Transformation of American Medicine. New York: Basic Books.

Struck M (1995) What OTs know that others don't. Advance for Occupational Therapists, 17 July: 4.

Swerdlow J (1999) Global culture. National Geographic 196(2), Aug.: 2–5.

Tracy SE (1918) Studies in Invalid Occupations: a Manual for Nurses and Attendants. Boston: Whitcomb & Barrows.

Tribute to Eleanor Clarke Slagle (1938) The Psychiatric Quarterly Supplement 12(1): 9–15.

Triggs OL (1902) Chapters in the History of the Arts and Crafts Movement. Chicago: Bohemia Guild of the Industrial Arts League.

von Bertalanffy L (1962) General Systems Theory. New York: George Braziller.

Voss DE, Ionta MK, Myers BJ (1985) Proprioceptive Neuromuscular Facilitation: Patterns and Techniques, 3rd edn. Philadelphia: Harper & Row.

White R (1963) Ego and reality in psychoanalytic theory. Psychoanalytic Issues 3. New York: International Universities Press.

White R (1971) The urge towards competence. American Journal of Occupational Therapy 25: 271–4.
Whitehead AN (1957) In P Medawar (ed.), The Uniqueness of the Individual. London: Methuen.
Winters E (ed.) (1952) The Collected Papers of Adolf Meyer (4 vols). Baltimore: Johns Hopkins Press.
Winters R (1998) Hooking up: computers are as much a part of campus life as football games and Lit lectures. Time/The Princeton Review, College Guide 2000: 21–2.
Wired for Success (1999) Seton Hall University's Mobile Computing Program starts students off with the right connections. Mobile Computing & Communications July: 103–5.
Yahoo Internet Life (2002) Retrieved April 24, 2002, from the World Wide Web: http://yil.com/features/feature.asp? Frame = false&Volume = 07&Issue = 1.
Yerxa EJ (1967) 1966 Eleanor Clarke Slagle Lecture: Authentic occupational therapy. American Journal of Occupational Therapy 21: 1–9.
Yerxa EJ (1979) The philosophical base of occupational therapy. In Occupational Therapy: 2001 A.D.: 26–30. Rockville, MD: American Occupational Therapy Association.

Index